Headache:
A MULTIMODAL PROGRAM FOR
Relief

C. David Tollison, Ph.D.
& Joseph W. Tollison, M.D.

Sterling Publishing Co., Inc. New York

To our Mother and Father.

All illustrations by Bonnie Adamson.

Library of Congress Cataloging in Publication Data

Tollison, C. David, 1949-
  Headache: a multimodal program for relief.

  Includes bibliographical references and index.
  1. Headache—Treatment. I. Tollison, Joseph W.
II. Title.
RC392.T64   1982   616.8'49   82-50550
ISBN 0-8069-5572-4
ISBN 0-8069-5573-2 (lib. bdg.)
ISBN 0-8069-7648-9 (pbk.)

Copyright © 1982 by Sterling Publishing Co., Inc.
Published by Sterling Publishing Co., Inc.
Two Park Avenue, New York, N.Y. 10016
Distributed in Australia by Oak Tree Press Co., Ltd.
P.O. Box K514 Haymarket, Sydney 2000, N.S.W.
Distributed in the United Kingdom by Blandford Press
Link House, West Street, Poole, Dorset BH15 1LL, England
Distributed in Canada by Oak Tree Press Ltd.
c/o Canadian Manda Group, 215 Lakeshore Boulevard East
Toronto, Ontario M5A 3W9
Manufactured in the United States of America
All rights reserved

Contents

Acknowledgments

Many individuals have contributed to this book, and we are pleased to acknowledge their assistance and support. Ms. Rose-Marie Strassberg of Sterling Publishing Company extensively edited and contributed constructive comments regarding style and presentation for which we are most grateful. Mrs. Tina Miller, Mrs. Dianne Massey and Mrs. Wilma Forbes greatly facilitated the preparation of this book by their unflagging and uncomplaining efforts in typing various portions of the manuscript. Dr. William D. Taylor offered constructive suggestions and comments on Chapter 5 which we found very valuable and helpful.

We would like to acknowledge our appreciation to our families for their support. To Linda, Courtney and David, and to Betty, Joey and Julie, we say thank you.

Preface

It comes as no surprise that numerous books have been written about head pain. The most prevalent of all human diseases, headaches strike 70 to 80 percent of the world's population at least once a month. Of those suffering more frequent headaches, over 15 million people in the United States are believed to suffer from migraine, the most painful of all headaches, while another 25 million Americans are afflicted with chronic "tension" or muscle-contraction headaches.* A survey of practically any bookstore is evidence of the public's interest and search for help in controlling this painful and common problem that too frequently resists the best efforts of traditional medical treatment. However, most of the books on head pain devote chapter after chapter to detailed descriptions of headache types and symptoms, yet offer little specific information to answer the one question that all headache sufferers ask: What can be done to remedy headache pain?

Headache: A Multimodal Program for Relief is different. Written for the reader who has no medical training but who wishes to learn to control headache pain, this text outlines specific steps to involve the headache victim in eliminating, or at least reducing, the frequency and intensity of headache pain. *Headache: A Multimodal Program for Relief* describes three major areas, which are: (1) Understanding Head Pain, (2) Traditional Headache Treatment and (3) A Multimodal

*H. Gould, *Headaches and Health* (New York: St. Martins Press, 1973), p. 23.

Program for Headache Relief. The program outlined in this book is not intended to substitute for the important role of medical care. Rather, it is designed to complement medical treatment and to educate and actively involve the headache sufferer in his or her own treatment. Research has indicated that the patient who is educated and involved in his or her health care is more likely to benefit from treatment.

A comprehensive multimodal program for headache relief is specifically outlined. Some therapies require the assistance of a doctor, while others can be done by the patient at home. This book describes the more traditional medical approaches to headache treatment, ranging from the common (medications) to the uncommon (surgery), giving primary emphasis to new and interesting techniques of pain relief that are currently receiving much public and professional attention. Massage, relaxation, hypnosis, dietary control, biofeedback and physical conditioning, combined in a comprehensive treatment program, offer a supplemental management program for headache sufferers whose pain has not adequately responded to conventional treatment. By combining detailed descriptions of traditional medical treatments with novel techniques to actively involve the sufferer in his or her own health care, *Headache: A Multimodal Program for Relief* represents an innovative and informative guide to eliminating the agony of headache pain. Particularly interesting to the many millions of people who suffer two or more disabling headaches each month, this book outlines a new approach to eliminating headaches. At long last there is help for millions of headache sufferers whose pain has not responded to traditional health care!

1

The History of Head Pain

Are headaches a symptom of our contemporary fast-paced and stressful life-styles? The answer is both yes and no. The incidence of headache does seem to increase with mounting stress factors common in modern society. The same may be said for other disorders thought to be stress-related, such as coronary artery disease and certain types of ulcers and emotional disorders. Yet headaches have plagued mankind for thousands of years, afflicting generations of our ancestors with the same intense agony and distress that many of us suffer today.

We know that primitive man believed that head pain was the work of evil spirits who invaded the body of unfortunate individuals. Well-intentioned early medical men set about to resolve the suffering of their patients in a most logical manner. If headache was caused by the invasion of evil spirits, then letting the spirits out of the skull should bring relief; thus was born a surgical procedure known as trepanning. Early medical men would solicit the aid of several strong assistants to hold the patient down, while some sharp object was used to bore a hole in the skull of the headache sufferer to let out evil spirits. In primitive Melanesian colonies on an island in the South Pacific, the custom of trepanning was a popular treatment for insanity, epilepsy and persistent headaches. Skulls showing signs of trepanning have been found in Europe and on the North and South

American continents, particularly in Mexico and Peru, dating back to the Neolithic and Bronze Ages. The skulls found in Europe have oval openings with edges that appear to be partially healed. This would indicate that the patient had surprisingly survived the surgery for some time. If we accept these trepanned skulls as evidence of headache-relief surgery, then the history of headache extends back ten thousand years or more.

Even if we limit ourselves to written accounts, headache still has a history of respectable antiquity: The earliest medical records of many ancient cultures make reference to it. Headache is mentioned in the *Atharvaveda* of India, a book on the knowledge of magic formulas that was written between 1500 and 800 B.C.

From the Babylonian era comes an interesting and poetic reference to headache which is believed to date from 4000 to 3000 B.C.*

Headache roameth over the desert, blowing like the wind,
Flashing like lightning, it is loosed above and below;
It cutteth off him who feareth not his god like a reed,
Like a stalk of henna it slitteth his thews,
It wasteth the flesh of him who hath no protecting goddess,
Flashing like a heavenly star, it cometh like the dew;
It standeth hostile against the wayfarer, scorching him like
    the day,
This man it hath struck and
Like one with heart disease he staggereth,
Like one bereft of reason he is broken,
Like that which has been cast into the fire he is shrivelled,
Like a wild ass . . . his eyes are full of cloud,
On himself he feedeth, bound in death;
Headache whose course like the dread windstorm none
    knoweth,
None knoweth its full time or its bond.

Ebers Papyrus, trans. W. R. Dawson, as cited by J. W. Lance, *Headache* (New York: Charles Scribner and Sons, 1975), p. 4.

A detailed description of migraine was submitted by Aretaeus, a physician born in Cappadocia in Asia Minor (now part of Turkey) who practiced in Alexandria, about 81 A.D. He emphasized that migraine pain frequently affects one side of the head and named this headache pain heterocrania. His description of headache pain is as follows:

> In certain cases the parts on the right side, or those on the left solely, so far that a separate temple, or ear, or one eyebrow, or one eye, or the nose which divides the face into two equal parts; and the pain does not pass this limit, but remains in the half of the head. This is called heterocrania, an illness by no means mild, even though it intermits, and although it appears to be slight. For if at any time it sets in acutely, it occasions unseemly and dreadful symptoms, spasm and distortion of the countenance takes place; the eyes either fixed intently like horns, or they are rolled inwardly to this side or to that; vertigo, deep-seated pain of the eyes as far as the meninges; irrestrainable sweat; sudden pain of the tendons, as of one striking with a club; nausea, vomiting of bilious matters; collapse of the patient... there is much torpor, heaviness of the head, anxiety and ennui. For they flee the light; the darkness soothes their disease: nor can they bear readily to look upon or hear anything agreeable; their sense of smell is vitiated, neither does anything agreeable to smell delight them, and they have also an aversion to fetid things: the patients, moreover, are weary of life, and wish to die.*

Galen (131 to 200 A.D., a Greek physician and writer), later called one-sided headache hemicrania, this term being the origin of the Old English word *megrim* and the French word *migraine.*

In 600 A.D., Paul of Aegina, a Greek physician at the

*Adams, F., *The Extant Works of Aretaeus, the Cappadocian,* cited by J. W. Lance, *Headache* (New York: Charles Scribner and Sons, 1975), p. 7.

Medical School of Alexandria, wrote: "Headache, which is one of the most serious complaints, is sometimes occasioned by an intemperament solely; sometimes by a redundance of humors, and sometimes by both." This idea was in keeping with the early Greek medical concept of four humors which were thought to govern health and disease—blood, phlegm, yellow bile and black bile. Over the centuries, these four humors came to be known as the types of "temperaments"— sanguine, phlegmatic, melancholic and choleric.

The nineteenth century brought in the Golden Age of description and classification in medicine, although it must be said that treatment modes remained firmly in the Dark Ages.

Today, medication is a primary treatment modality for headache, but the use of medication to combat headache pain is not a new concept. In a ritual used by Cherokee Indian medicine men, the headache patient chewed ginseng, the root of a plant with reported medicinal properties, while the forehead was rubbed gently with the palm of the right hand and a mixture of water and ginseng juice was sprinkled over the painful area. It would seem that in selected cases, the relief obtained from this primitive Cherokee therapy approaches that of modern ergotamine preparations (Chapter 5), but would have far fewer negative side effects.

Acupuncture is presently receiving much serious study because of recent reports of its efficacy in relieving headache and other pain. Acupuncture has been used in traditional Chinese medicine since it was devised by Huang Ti, who was said to have lived from 2698 to 2598 B.C.

With all of the sophistication of modern health care, have we won the war against headache? Unfortunately, the answer is no. Despite complex pharmacologic agents, 10 to 12 percent of the American population continues suffering the agony of recurrent head pain. Perhaps it is now time to reexamine our approach to headache treatment. Perhaps it is time to consider an innovative approach to supplement headache treatment that, on closer examination, is really not new at all. Perhaps it is time to "get back to the basics," without throwing away the advances of modern medical care, yet actively involving the patient in the care of his own body. The following anecdote* may serve as a fitting conclusion to this brief historical review and as an introduction to the remainder of this text as well:

> About once a month, until the age of 70, George Bernard Shaw suffered a devastating headache which lasted for a day. One afternoon, after recovering from an attack, he was introduced to Nansen and asked the famous Arctic explorer whether he had ever discovered a headache cure.
> "No," said Nansen with a look of amazement.
> "Have you ever tried to find a cure for headaches?"
> "No."
> "Well, that is a most astonishing thing!" exclaimed Shaw. "You have spent your life in trying to discover the North Pole, which nobody on earth cares tuppence about, and you have never attempted to discover a cure for the headache, which every living person is crying aloud for."

*W. G. Lennox and M. A. Lennox, *Epilepsy and Related Disorders*, Vol. I (London: Churchill, 1960), p. 216.

2

Why Headaches Hurt

It may be surprising to learn that headache pain *does not* come from your brain. Curiously enough, the brain itself is relatively insensitive to pain. In fact, some brain surgeries can be performed while the patient is wide awake. If the surface of your brain, the cortex, is touched or stimulated by an electrical current, you may feel a tingling down the opposite side of the body, see flashes of light in front of your eyes, or experience other sensations in the part of the brain which is stimulated. You will not, however, feel pain, even if your brain tissue is cut with a scalpel. Generally speaking, pain from the head and neck comes from nerves supplying various arteries and muscles. If we are to fully understand why headaches hurt, a general knowledge of the structure and organization of the head and neck is essential.

"HEADACHE" VESSELS

Veins and arteries—the conduits of the bloodstream—are very flexible structures. They dilate and constrict in response to changes in body chemistry and muscle contraction. Their diameters change constantly throughout the course of a day. It is only when they become overly swollen that some form of discomfort results.

The chief artery of interest to many headache sufferers is the temporal artery, especially the so-called superficial branch. This artery ascends on both sides of the head from the neck, below and in front of the ears, upward directly in front of the ears, and then angles forward and upward to the upper temple area. From the temple area, the artery divides widely over the forehead (Figure 2-1). The temporal artery is involved in a large percentage of headaches.

The second most important artery is the occipital artery. This artery arises from beneath and behind the ears on each side of the head and divides inward from each side across the lower back of the skull (Figure 2-1).

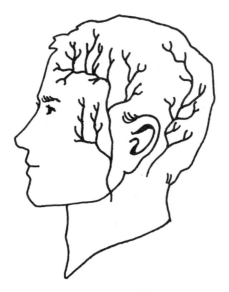

Figure 2-1: Occipital and cranial arteries

The temporal and occipital arteries assist in supplying blood and oxygen to the brain (oxygen is transported to the brain via red blood cells). The brain requires a generous flow of blood and oxygen to function effectively and, in fact, uses more than 25 percent of the body's supply of blood. Arteries transport blood throughout the brain while veins take the deoxygenated blood away. We cannot exist if the blood and its precious cargo of oxygen are denied the brain for longer than minutes. Cerebral circulation is certainly one of the body's most crucial processes, and the temporal and occipital arteries play an important role.

Headaches occur when certain blood vessels in the head (frequently the temporal and occipital arteries) dilate and impinge on the pain-sensitive cranial nerves. The presence of some dilated, headache-causing blood vessels can be detected with the naked eye. The superficial temporal artery, located at the side of the temples, can be felt as a steady pulse during normal moments, but during a headache this pulse becomes a heavy throb, so intense that the pulsating artery is occasionally visible on the forehead. Many more vessels invisible to the naked eye have been studied with the use of radioactive gases that trace circulation and with X rays taken with high-contrast fluid. Researchers have documented remarkable changes in the rate of circulation and vascular diameter during a headache. The dilated vessels press the nerve endings which send messages of pain to the brain. Many responses then occur in the system to restore equilibrium, but the only phenomenon that penetrates to the consciousness of the sufferer is pain.

Headache victims can feel the changes often associated with headache taking place in their bodies. The feeling of dread and depression which often heralds a headache is caused by the fluctuations of the blood vessels and their effects on the emotions. The relentless throbbing frequently associated with vascular headaches is caused by the pulsation of arteries engorged with blood. Fluid will flow through a tube at a rate determined by the fourth power of its radius, meaning that when artery walls are only slightly distended, the volume and acceleration of blood is greatly increased.

Blood circulation is subject to many influences within the body: The deep flush of an intoxicated man and the delicate blush of a young woman, for example, are similar in character, if not in etiology. Though the cause may be quite different, the quality or color of the flush may be remarkably similar. Circulation is psychophysical: It may be caused by organic or psychological stimuli. It is no wonder then that our blood will go pounding through the arteries of our head at the slightest disturbance, whether the disturbance is organic or psychological in nature or is a combination of the two. When this occurs, pain-sensitive nerves are stimulated and the agony of a headache soon follows.

"HEADACHE" MUSCLES

Muscles located in the neck and head and considered suspect in the etiology of certain types of headaches can be divided, like the "headache arteries," into front and rear groups. In the frontal group, although actually located on the side of the head, is the temporalis muscle. This muscle covers a wide area along the side of the head and attaches to the lower jaw (Figure 2-2). Place your fingertips in a straight line between the top of your ear and your eyebrow and clench your teeth tightly. The movement your fingers detect is the temporalis muscle. During stressful situations, many of us have a tendency to tighten the jaw and the temporalis muscle.

The frontalis muscle covers the front of the head and forehead like a cap, and it is frequently involved in muscle-contraction headaches (Figure 2-3). This important muscle raises the eyebrows and moves the scalp forward. The frontalis is often targeted as a prime muscle for biofeedback treatment. Frontalis tension is common during stressful periods and can result in chronic headaches.

The back of the head is also frequently the site of headaches because of the occipitalis muscle. The occipitalis is a

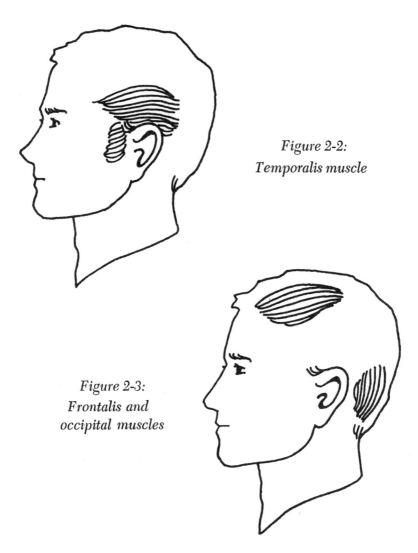

Figure 2-2:
Temporalis muscle

Figure 2-3:
Frontalis and
occipital muscles

key headache muscle because of its strategic location at the lower back of the skull and because the occipital artery lies embedded in it (Figure 2-3). Of most importance is a wide group of muscles that connect the rear base of the head with several of the cervical (neck) vertebrae of the spinal column. These muscles cross over and support each other in action as they flex, rotate and hold the head. One of these smaller muscles also connects to your shoulder blades.

Overlying all these is probably the single most important muscle in tension headaches: the trapezius (Figure 2-4). This strong and larger muscle gives our shoulders much of their shape. Notice on Figure 2-4 that the origin of the trapezius is the external occipital protuberance. To locate the protuberance on either side of the head, place the index finger of each hand directly behind each ear. Here you should feel a rounded knob that is located an inch or two to each side of the midline. Those are the protuberances, and they are very important to your headaches, not in themselves

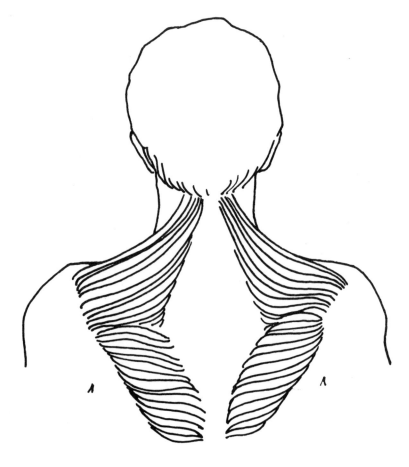

Figure 2-4: Trapezius muscle

(skull bones do not cause headaches), but because of the trapezius muscle that is attached to them. The area from these bones to the top of your shoulder blades is a very important area for muscle-contraction headaches, by far the most common form of headache, and may even be involved to some extent in migraines.

You will note from Figure 2-4 that the trapezius is triangular, with the broad base of the triangle running up along the spine. The middle and lower parts of the muscle originate along the spinal verterbrae and cross over to the shoulder blade where the muscle attaches at the shoulder. These parts are frequently involved in tension felt in the back and shoulders, but the prime culprit in headaches is the upper section, running from the skull to the shoulder blade. Shrug your shoulders and you can feel this muscle tense and lift the shoulders. Locking the shoulders in position and then tensing them will pull the head back. Many shoulder and neck motions are emphasized in the chapters on manipulation and massage (Chapter 8), relaxation exercises (Chapter 9), and physical conditioning (Chapter 11), as part of a multimodal program for headache relief.

"HEADACHE" NERVES

It is important to remember that pain exists *only* if it is perceived. For example, a paraplegic may sit by a fireplace engaged in casual conversation, totally unaware that the fire is causing a traumatic and serious burn to his leg. Why? Paraplegics have suffered a spinal cord injury that essentially blocks the transmission of nerve impulses from the legs to the brain. Not only are they paralyzed, but pain sensations from the lower-half of the body are not registered in the brain. The nerves serve as "highways" or "telephone lines" from the transmission of pain messages to the brain.

Pain sensations are carried by two different types of nerve fibres. Immediately after a traumatic or chemical disruption in the body, the so-called "A" fibres speed the news of this occurrence to the central nervous system and the brain. The "A" fibres transmit messages at the speed of approximately 300 feet per second. They pinpoint the affected area with a sharp, well-localized pain. Meanwhile, this same pain message has been picked up by the "C" fibres, which are much smaller than the "A" fibres. In addition, the "C" fibres travel at a much slower rate, a speed of about three feet per second. By the time their message arrives at the brain, it has already been received by the "A" fibres. The nervous system, brain and the consciousness have been alerted to the message of pain, and steps to correct the situation are being planned by all three. But the "C" fibres continue their thankless task, laboriously transmitting this unwanted signal, which is now manifested as a dull, throbbing ache.

The different pain messages are easily discerned after a minor household accident, a cut or bump on the head. The first sensation is sharp, shocking, momentarily unbearable. You would likely go into shock if the pain from the initial trauma continued at that intensity. Fortunately, the tortoise-like "C" fibres carry a more tolerable message. The transmission of pain messages during a headache is constant. As long as muscles are tensed or arteries are dilated and pressing on nerves, there is pain. The nervous system, brain and the consciousness must deal with an endless procession of nerve impulses that tell them something they've known for hours, forcing them to act when their actions serve only to worsen the situation.

One of the larger nerves, which serves much of the area of the face and front two-thirds of the scalp, is the fifth cranial or trigeminal nerve (Figure 2-5). This nerve gets its name because it has three major divisions. (The Latin *trigeminus* means "three born together.") The trigeminal nerve has branches that travel to facial skin, part of the scalp, mucous membranes of the mouth and nasal cavity, eyes, teeth and *dura mater* of the brain. If this nerve is irritated, it causes pain in the forehead, cheek or jaw, depending on which of the three branches is involved. For example, if sinuses in the forehead are inflamed, the swollen lining of the sinuses presses against the fine nerve branches embedded there. The pressure triggers the transmission of nerve impulses which travel along the first division of the trigeminal nerve. If the maxillary sinuses in the cheekbones or a tooth in the upper jaw become inflamed, pain signals travel along the second division. If a tooth in the lower jaw or the jawbone itself is the cause of the trouble, pain impulses travel along the third division.

The three divisions join together inside the skull where their combined fibres enter the brain stem, which lies under the brain like the stalk of a mushroom. Some fibres pass directly upward into the brain itself, while others make a loop

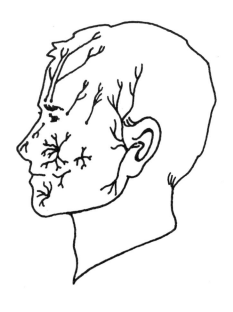

Figure 2-5:
Trigeminal nerve
distribution

downward into the upper part of the spinal cord. This loop is very important in understanding head and neck pain because it connects with the same nerve cells that receive impulses from the upper part of the neck. For this reason, a disturbance of the bones or discs in the upper part of the head and neck can cause pain to be felt in other parts of the body, a phenomenon known as referred pain. When this pathway is operating in the reverse direction, a headache such as migraine can be accompanied by severe pain and stiffness in the neck.

In addition to supplying the face and skull with pain sensation, the trigeminal nerve is responsible for picking up sensations from the blood vessels in the brain and scalp. When blood vessels dilate, the trigeminal nerve is there to quickly rush the message of a painful vascular headache to the brain. When an artery becomes distended, the delicate network of nerve fibres around it stretches and gives off signals which may increase with each pulse, so the headache may be described as throbbing. If you press your finger firmly against the pulsating artery located in front of the ear, the pain will temporarily ease since less blood flows through the vessel with each pulse.

For our purposes, the following general rule of thumb may prove beneficial: Draw a straight line upward from the ear. Any head pain that you experience in front of that line probably results from activity in the trigeminal nerve. Any head pain behind that line results from the spinal nerves which run down over the back of the head to join the upper part of the spinal cord.

Now that we have reviewed the anatomical and physiological structures involved in headaches, let's take a look at the product of headache: *pain*. In the next chapter we will learn that pain is composed of at least two major components, organic processes and our psychological response.

3

Understanding Pain

Before the early part of the nineteenth century, the phenomenon of pain was viewed as an essentially emotional event. This concept had for many centuries changed little from that expressed in the early dissertations of Aristotle, who considered pain in the category of an emotion—specifically, the opposite of pleasure. Aristotle believed that pain was more an appropriate topic for philosophical study than a consideration for physicians.

With the advances of science and the explosion of knowledge concerning the structure and function of the human body, neurophysiology and neurology increasingly challenged these philosophical ideas and ultimately succeeded in establishing the importance of considering pain a physiological phenomenon. Much interest has subsequently been generated in clarifying the nature of pain in physiological terms. While no theoretical model has yet been devised that can account for all the experimental and clinical observations concerning it, there is widespread agreement among researchers in the field of pain, especially chronic pain, that the phenomenon we call pain is much more complex than traditional physiological explanations would suggest. In fact . . . pain is today considered a complex subjective perception composed of at least *two* major components: physiology and psychology.

NOTE: Pages 23–33 are excerpted from *Managing Chronic Pain: A Patient's Guide* by C. David Tollison, Ph.D. (New York: Sterling Publishing Co., 1982), pp. 16–25.

PHYSIOLOGICAL MECHANISMS OF PAIN

Physiological Structure and Function

The perception of pain involves the entire central nervous system: the brain, spinal cord and miles of nerves in the body. The central nervous system controls the *voluntary* muscles such as those used in walking, picking up a pencil, combing your hair and playing tennis. The phenomenon of pain also involves the sympathetic nervous system, a part of the autonomic nervous system. The autonomic nervous system controls the "automatic," or *involuntary* muscles such as the heart muscle and the muscles that dilate and contract the pupils in your eyes. The sympathetic nerves travel to all the arteries in the body which, in turn, control the amount of blood flow to the muscles.

Nerves serve an important function in the body since they act as pain perceptors, picking up pain messages much as a radio antenna picks up radio waves. Pain begins as a stimulus, which is then picked up by nerves. Once a pain stimulus or message is received by a nerve ending, it is carried to the brain and back again to the affected body part by the nerves. Some nerves are single strands of fibre while others are bundled together. Some nerves are coated with a substance called myelin while others are not. Myelin acts as a protective insulation for the electrical charges of nerves.

Nerves are made up of tiny nerve cells which receive and forward pain messages. Each cell has a receiver end called a dendrite and a transmitter end called an axon. Pain messages travel as an electrical impulse from the axons of one cell to the dendrites of the next, and so on down the line. The gap between the axons and dendrites is called a synapse, and it is here that pain messages are deciphered and coded. Depending on the type of coding, a pain message reaching a synapse may be terminated completely, changed and re-

24

routed in some way, or simply forwarded to the neighboring cell.

This "decision at the synapse" is influenced strongly by chemical substances called neurotransmitters that are activated by pain messages. Neurotransmitters also assist in the pain–message transmission since they "bridge the gap" between axons and dendrites. A number of different neurotransmitters have been identified, including serotonin, dopamine, norepinephrine and acetylcholine. This transmission process, however, can be reduced or increased by drugs. In fact, many drugs are purposely designed to alter the transmission of electrical impulses across the synapse.

Many researchers believe that pain messages travel to the brain on one of two "superhighways." The pain message starts with a stimulus and travels up the spinal cord. This highway is called the spinothalamic tract. Once the message gets to the brain, it meets a fork in the road. One highway travels through portions of the brain called the thalamus and hypothalamus to the limbic system. This highway is called the paleospinothalamic tract. This is the tract on which pain that's been described as a steady-ache or dull-ache travels. The other highway is called the neospinothalamic tract. Sharp, stabbing impulses usually travel this highway to the brain.

Biochemistry of Pain

A current topic of interest and debate in scientific circles is the role of biological chemicals in the experience of pain. Unfortunately, there exists much theory, but little fact. In the past few years, most investigative efforts have focussed on the importance of protein substances called neurokinins and the role they play in reducing pain thresholds. Many researchers believe that the experience of pain triggers the release of neurokinins in the body, increasing the discomforting quality of pain. A simple way to think of the role of neurokinins is to imagine a dam and a reservoir. Under most conditions, neurokinins are safely stored in the body much like water backed up by a dam. However, under certain conditions, such as heavy and prolonged rain, the dam can break, causing flooding and greatly complicating a bad situation. When pain is experienced, there is not only the problem of discomfort, but the pain may "break the dam" and release a flood of neurokinins, which in turn increase the pain.

One neurokinin theory postulates that the substances are released when tissue cells are damaged or destroyed. The release of neurokinins then concentrates around nerve endings and fibres involved in the transmission of pain signals from a body part to the brain. As the pain message travels up a nerve, neurokinins "amplify" the pain signal.

A similar process has been known to occur in migraine headaches. In the early stage of migraine development, another biochemical, serotonin, is released in the body. Serotonin causes vasoconstriction (arteries in the head decrease their diameter and allow less blood flow). Constriction of the cephalic arteries (located in the head area) and decreased blood flow is thought by many researchers to cause the "flashing lights" and uneasy, light-headed feeling known as prodromals that many migraine victims suffer prior to the onset of severe pain. Once the serotonin is depleted, however, the arteries become more flexible, the body is flooded with a release of neurokinins, and the arteries dilate in throbbing, excruciating pain. The presence of neurokinins is thought to lower the threshold at which the throbbing arterial dilations are felt as painful.

The Endorphins

Not only does the body manufacture biochemicals that

amplify the intensity of pain (such as neurokinins), but recent research has also identified pain-reducing biochemicals produced in the human body. The name given to these substances is endorphins, and many researchers believe they represent an important component of the body's own mechanism for controlling pain.

Endorphins have a number of similarities to potent narcotic analgesic drugs such as morphine. . . . For example, endorphins are nearly identical to morphine in molecular structure. In addition, endorphins, like morphine, exert their chemical action by blocking a number of important transmission sites in the central nervous system. This alteration in nerve transmission seems to decrease the intensity and quality of pain. Finally, endorphins are thought to act on the same special cells in the brain and spinal cord that the opiate narcotic drugs attach to in order to produce an analgesic and euphoric effect. Commonly known as opiate receptor cells, these cells seem to have a special affinity for man-made narcotic drugs. This affinity has led researchers to suspect the existence of endorphins even before they were formally identified.

If you seem to have a lower threshold for pain than other people, perhaps your body has a deficiency of endorphins or receptor cells. Research in this area is continuing to document the important role of endorphins in the experience of pain. Endorphins may be prescribed someday to treat chronic pain, depression and other related disorders. To harness the human body's pain-reducing chemicals for use in treating medical disorders would solve a giant portion of the puzzle of pain.

Gate Control Theory

In 1965, Drs. Ronald Melzack and Patrick Wall* proposed

*Dr. Melzack is a psychologist; Dr. Wall is a neuroanatomist.

a theory to explain how pain messages travel up the spinal cord to the brain. While the accuracy of this theory remains a topic of debate, there is little doubt that their theory, known as the Gate Control Theory, represents the single most important theoretical contribution to the field of pain research.

The gate theory suggests that a specialized group of nerve cells in the substantia gelatinosa (located in the butterfly-shaped portion of the spinal cord known as the dorsal horn) acts as a control mechanism similar to a valve or gate. The gate regulates the flow of pain messages into the central nervous system from peripheral nerves. When the gate is open, pain messages pass through to the brain and register pain. When the gate is closed, pain messages do not pass through and, theoretically, pain should not be experienced.

According to Drs. Melzack and Wall, small bundles of nerve fibre keep the gate open, and larger nerve-fibre bundles, whose messages travel faster than messages on the smaller bundles, can close the gate. Accordingly, if you pinch your finger in a desk drawer, the pain will slowly travel up small nerve-fibre bundles towards the brain. If you briskly rub your finger and hand, the response of rubbing will initiate a faster message along large nerve-fibre bundles, signalling the gate to close and limiting the amount of pain you experience.

Psychological variables also play a role in regulating the flow of pain messages through the gate. We may closely attend to the pain or use distraction techniques to keep our mind off pain. In addition, the expectation and stress of pain have an impact on the function of the gate.

PSYCHOLOGICAL MECHANISMS OF PAIN

Personality and Pain

Perhaps half of the distressing quality of chronic pain is

psychological. This is not to say that half of all chronic-pain patients experience pain that is psychological in origin. Although pain that results from mental and emotional causes (psychogenic pain) is very real, it affects only a small portion of the patients who suffer chronic [or recurrent pain]. A far more common occurrence is . . . pain that began with some physical injury or disorder.

When a victim is forced to deal with unrelenting pain for days, weeks, months and even years, the most stalwart and stable mind can falter. Chronic pain changes any sufferer's personality to some extent and some individuals lose their ability to respond to their surroundings. We may concentrate less on interpersonal relationships than on the pain itself. Relationships then become troublesome rather than joyful. As the distress is prolonged over months, we may become withdrawn, moody, irritable and eventually depressed to the point where life's goals and responsibilities are forsaken.

Personality changes wrought by the persistence of pain are thought by some scientists to be rooted in anatomical connections between deep-seated pain reception centers in the thalamus of the brain and the frontal lobes of the cerebral hemispheres. The frontal lobes, in general, serve human conscious effort in directing day-to-day activities and planning long- and short-term events. The nerve centers of the frontal lobes must receive information from the environment surrounding the body, and the sensory nervous system supplies this information. Nerve fibre bundles then relay this information to areas of the brain where data from previous experiences is stored. Under ordinary circumstances, the process continues until a goal or set of goals is formulated. Then the brain motor systems are engaged to carry out the planned process.

When new, incoming sensory information is experienced as painful, either because a pain message from a body part is received or because the sensory element is unpleasant as compared with prior experiences, the frontal lobe system of the brain becomes dominated by the incoming stimulus or stimuli. Our attention is then continuously diverted to the painful sensation. The painful stimulus is thought to interfere with our normal conscious thought processes. If a painful stimulus persists, a consistent, conscious effort and a great deal of mental energy are required to divert our attention away from the pain. If the pain is relatively mild, energy is easily replenished, and consciousness is easily directed as our will desires. However, when the painful stimulus is of high intensity, the psychological energy demands are great, fatigue sets in, and our conscious attention is drawn more and more to the painful problem.

This overview of how personality and mental processes become involved in the experience of chronic pain is an obvious oversimplification of brain mechanisms and the complex interplay of physical and psychological variables. Numerous other factors such as fear, distraction, anxiety, depression, expectations and stress play important roles in shaping our perception of pain and influencing our ability either to effectively live with chronic pain or be controlled and disabled by it.

Less independent individuals, for example, often desire to be cared for by those around them. Many times, however, a dependency role is not possible, as in the case of heads of families. If such individuals wish relief from their roles as supporters and leaders, [a headache or other type of pain problem] can satisfy a secret desire for dependence, without the embarrassment of an open admission. A mild pain is magnified or the symptoms of a cured disorder are prolonged. The patient, consciously or unconsciously, needs pain to satisfy long-standing emotional needs.

A similar situation can exist with chronic-pain victims

whose premorbid personality (personality prior to the onset of pain) is marked by dissatisfaction and unhappiness. Perhaps discontent is the result of a boring career, advanced age, marital dissatisfaction or family role. To a person "trapped" in one of these unpleasant situations, even daily tasks become drudgery. [A headache problem] may provide the excuse to cease performing burdensome tasks and, because of the sympathy of family and friends, the victim can still maintain a respected role in the eyes of others.

Expectations and Pain

A simple suspicion that has recently been verified experimentally is this: If you expect something to hurt, it probably will. Again, we emphasize the complex relationship between the mind and body. This relationship is so complex and the interplay of psychological and physical variables so confounded, that to fully explain or separate the mind from the body is an impossible task. Consider, for example, this 1889 medical report from Dr. C. Lloyd Tuckey, a physician.

There are few cases of this kind more remarkable than one related by Mr. Woodhouse Braine, the well-known chloroformist. Having to administer ether to an hysterical girl who was about to be operated on for the removal of two sebaceous tumors from the scalp, he found that the ether bottle was empty, and that the inhaling bag was free from even the odor of any anesthetic. While a fresh supply was being obtained, he thought to familiarize the patient with the process by putting the inhaling bag over her mouth and nose, and telling her to breathe quietly and deeply. After a few inspirations, she cried "Oh, I feel it; I am going off," and a moment after, her eyes turned up, and she became unconscious. As she was found to be perfectly insensible and the ether had not yet come, Mr. Braine proposed that the surgeon should proceed with the operation. One tumor was removed without in the least disturbing her, and then, in order to test her condition, a bystander said that she was coming to. Upon this she began to show signs of waking, so the bag was once more applied, with the remark, "She'll soon be off again," when she immediately lost sensation and the operation was successfully and painlessly completed.*

Further substantiating the powerful influence of expectation in our experience is the phenomenon of placebo drugs. Placebos are usually plain salt or sugar pills with no active ingredients, yet the placebo effect on pain is often remarkable. Patients taking placebos are given the suggestion that they are powerful and effective drugs. For many pain patients, the expectation of relief produces pain relief that approaches the effectiveness of powerful analgesic drugs.

The role of pain intensity and expectation can also have an opposite effect. In one study, subjects were given two separate electrical shocks. Before each shock, subjects were given a description of what was to occur. The first description did not include the word "pain" or "painful" while the second description did. As you might guess, the second shock was consistently rated as more painful than the first even though the intensity of the electrical shocks was the same.

In cases of [headache] pain, it is the chronic, never-ending nature of the disease that alters our expectations. The depression and frustration of living in constant distress can soon deplete our optimism and expectations for relief. In time, we come to expect pain, and as our expectation of pain increases, so too does our pain. It soon becomes a cycle—the more we hurt, the more we expect to hurt; the more we expect to hurt, the more we hurt, and so on. Breaking the cycle of pain and expectation requires a determined and consistent effort. . . .

*M. Feuerstein & E. Skjei, *Mastering Pain* (New York: Bantam Books, 1979), p. 34.

Stress and Pain

In recent years emotional stress has been linked to a variety of physical disorders. A sampling of some of these disorders includes bronchial asthma, cardiovascular disease, obesity, gastrointestinal disorders (such as peptic ulcers) . . . dermatological disorders (such as neurodermatitis) and, of course, [headaches]. The effects of stress on pain appear to be three-fold. First, emotional stress can precipitate a physical disorder, such as muscle-contraction headaches . . . and certain types of cardiovascular disorders. Second, stress can deplete your body of the "psychological energy" required to cope effectively with chronic pain on a daily basis. Third, emotional stress can intensify already existing pain since stress is associated with muscle tension, fatigue and pain.

Dr. Beverly J. Volicer recently reported an interesting investigation of the relationship between stress and pain.* The results of this study suggest that reducing hospital stress can result in less analgesic drug use, reduced hospital stay and less pain. Conversely, high stress and anxiety levels resulted in increased pain and more numerous difficulties with digestion, mood and sleep.

The Headache Personality

Consider the case of Joan H., a successful public relations representative for a major industry. Joan is in her late thirties and has suffered from migraine headaches since she was fifteen years old. For almost twenty-five years she had had one or two severe headache attacks a week. Her vision would become blurred, and she would occasionally experience near-total blindness in her left eye. Nausea would well up inside

*Beverly J. Volicer, [M.D.], "Hospital Stress and Patient Reports of Pain," *Journal of Human Stress*, June 1978, pp. 28–37. Dr. Volicer is a psychiatrist.

of her, and violent, almost projectile vomiting would rack her body. The headache would rage incurably for several hours until it gradually subsided to a heavy dull ache. Her few pain-free hours were spent in dreadful anticipation of the next attack.

The migraine attacks came at all the predictable times: after an important meeting with a client, before or during vacation and frequently on weekends. During this time, Joan climbed steadily up the corporate ladder, raised a family, and from all external signs, lived a happy and successful life.

But Joan H. lived a double life, of which even her husband and family were not aware. She lived with pain, the dreaded anticipation of it and its aftermath. While underplaying her affliction to family, friends and colleagues, she was desperate for a cure. Or was she? It's true that she visited scores of doctors who performed various diagnostic tests. It is also true that at one point in her life the headaches became so bad that she seriously considered suicide to escape the devastating pain. But somehow she never managed to fully cooperate or complete any of the treatments she was offered. The potent pain relievers made her drowsy; tranquillizers dulled her mental functioning; antimigraine medication left her nervous and upset her stomach; eliminating cigarette and alcohol-consumption seemed too pat a remedy; psychotherapy was a waste of time; diet therapy was a useless fad; biofeedback was considered "weird"; and physical exercise took so much time, not to mention making her tired and sweaty.

Joan's major problem was simple: She did not want to be cured. For some inexplicable reason, she needed the pain and, according to many doctors and researchers, Joan has a good deal of company. Some researchers believe in the existence of a "migraine personality," described as a person whose desire for relief is questionable. Although they go through the motions of seeking medical help, they don't always follow the advice that is given them.

Migraine personality patients are also described as dealing with their lives in a way that rapidly depletes the reserve of energy. Typically, these personalities are thought to have been prevented from expressing normal aggressive feelings because of rigid parental attitudes. These persons are thought to have been pushed to perform beyond their capacity, thus increasing their feeling of inadequacy and frustration. The result is a headache victim. All the repressed rage and hostile feelings that are denied expression come out in the form of a headache. The victim simultaneously airs the forbidden feelings and punishes himself for having them.

Does the migraine personality really exist? Are all headache sufferers intelligent, ambitious, rigid, organized, cautious and emotionally repressed perfectionists? In our clinical experience, the answer is a resounding no. It is true that this personality type frequently suffers headaches, but the converse is equally true.

4

Causes and Types of Headaches

No animal suffers the torments of the human being. From hangnails to terminal diseases, from simple anxiety to complex and mysterious psychoses, humans spend more of their lives in physical and mental anguish than any other earthly creature.

Headaches are a prime example. Although statistics are difficult to compile, many researchers believe that at least seven out of ten people get at least one painful headache a month. What triggers headache? It is difficult to say. Not all headaches are located in the same part of the head, nor do they all occur for the same reasons or have the same symptoms.

MUSCLE-CONTRACTION (TENSION) HEADACHES

Over 90 percent of the people who suffer chronic headaches need never have them. They are not ill, and they have no special physical predisposition. On the surface there is nothing wrong with them, yet they suffer considerable discomfort. Their pain is real and excruciating, and is described in graphic terms as being like a tight band being wound around the forehead or a hammer beating inside the skull. Why is it that

NOTE: Pages 36–42 are excerpted from *Managing Chronic Pain: A Patient's Guide*, pp. 35–39.

these people, over 25 million in the United States alone, at a conservative count, are plagued in this manner? The answer is found in one deceptively simple word: tension.

Psychologically, the idea of tension is very complex, encompassing many different emotional states. But physiologically, it is easy to understand. The muscles are tense when they are prepared to take some action. [This kind of muscle set is called "bracing": The muscles prepare to freeze or to take a defensive position to avoid unpleasantness by having the important action muscles of the body ready to move or stand by. Considerable degrees of muscle tension, even "knots" can develop in the muscles.] To visualize this, you have only to flex the muscles in your arms or legs. This is their state during any physical exertion. If you keep the muscles in a state of tension without doing anything, you will soon begin to feel uncomfortable and will have to relax them after a while.

The mechanism of all tension headaches is a contraction of the muscles at the back of the head and neck above the shoulders [Figure 4-1]. The tensed muscles impinge upon the nerves that travel up the spinal column into the brain. The contraction also squeezes the blood vessels, following essentially the same path. This constriction of the blood vessels and irritation of the nerves lead to a headache. The action of the "headache muscles" is involuntary, but the act of contraction occurs for exactly the same reason that all the other muscles tense and relax. The headache muscles have gotten their signals crossed. They have been misled into anticipating an act of physical exertion and have needlessly prepared for it. Muscles can be said to "think" in that they often act independently of instructions from the brain. But they may not always think well. They may confuse neural messages, tensing at the wrong moment and maintaining tension when there is no reason to do so.

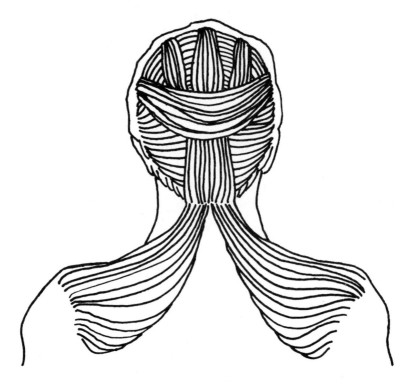

Figure 4-1: Contraction of "headache" muscles

The brain is an organ that has continually evolved with the development of the species—it did not exist in its present form in the first human creature. The thoughts and actions of early man were controlled from a point now known as the "old brain." The primitives led a very simple mental and emotional life. Their movements were dictated by elemental instincts and reflexes. [When frightened, the body prepared to defend itself. The muscles tensed, ready to fight, flee or freeze; the internal organs responded to ensure emergency functioning by increasing heart rate and blood pressure to give emergency supplies of blood and oxygen; digestion stopped and blood pooled where needed so the skin blanched. Today we experience many of these same physiological reactions when we are under stress or feel tense.

We also continue to] hunch our shoulders when caught in a rainstorm, although this gesture serves no purpose. Like a turtle retreating into its shell, we try to keep the hostile environment at bay.

What started as a reaction to immediate danger became a standard reflex withdrawal from all unpleasantness. As civilization became more complex, the stark terror of primeval man was replaced by a subtler type of fear known as anxiety. Where the primitives must have spent most of their lives cringing from the unknown, contemporary man knows very few moments of abject fear. We may go a whole lifetime without being afraid for our lives or facing any physical menace whatsoever. But very few of us can last a day without having at least one moment of anxiety.

The categories of anxiety are too numerous to detail. But in many people the body's reaction to all of them is the same. The "headache muscles" tighten up and remain tightened. Anxiety does not have the immediate quality of fear. It does not come and go quickly, but lingers on, giving the rest of the body plenty of time to react. It increases the secretion of certain hormones, some of which have an effect on the blood vessels. Adrenaline, the "fight or flight" hormone released when there is great stress or danger, also dribbles out in times of anxiety. The body acts as if it were in danger. There seems to be no communication between the primitive protective reflex and the part of the consciousness that deals with reality. [The result is frequently painful and recurring muscle-contraction headaches.]

MIGRAINE HEADACHES

About one out of every ten Americans suffers from migraine or vascular headaches. Though they affect fewer people than tension headaches do, migraines can be far more severe, disabling and difficult to treat.

Migraines are characterized by intense pain, usually located on one side of the head, and by a distinct throbbing sensation in the temples, like a pulse. [Twice as many women suffer migraine as men. Although it does occur in children, migraine most often strikes in the late teens or early twenties and continues until middle age, when it usually abates.] The victim may experience nausea, changes in vision (such as spots or geometric shapes in front of the eyes), temporary loss of vision, double vision, or sharply increased sensitivity to light just before and during a migraine attack. [These symptoms are thought to be caused by blood being shunted away from the cerebral cortex.]

Migrains tend to recur at [semi-regular] intervals: Most migraine victims can tell when an attack is imminent. Headaches may last for only a few hours, or for as long as two or three days. They may be so intense as to virtually incapacitate the victims, forcing the sufferer to do nothing but stay in bed in a quiet, darkened room. Many migraine victims report distinct mood changes just before and occasionally after a migraine attack, ranging from depression, irritability and confusion to elation and euphoria. Some report feeling a numbness in the opposite side of the body from the side of the head that hurts.

Researchers consider the causes of migraine to involve complex cycles of change in the body's vascular system. Factors such as sleep patterns, stress, genetic predisposition, hormone levels, allergies, weather patterns, fluid intake, and even ingredients in such common foods as chocolate, bananas, nuts, pork, red wine and certain cheeses have been implicated in the onset of certain kinds of migraine.

Experiments have shown that specific complex patterns of change in the circulation of blood in the head characterize the onset of migraine. The arteries constrict, then dilate. There are related biochemical changes, and there is a general increase in activity of the sympathetic nervous system.

This knowledge forms the theoretical framework for the current application of thermal biofeedback (Chapter 7) in the treatment of migraine headaches.

CLUSTER HEADACHES (MIGRAINOUS NEURALGIA)

Cluster headache is the only type of headache that primarily strikes men: Some 85 percent of all those affected by this type of headache are males. A curious intermittent pattern of bouts or clusters of intensely severe pains which recur once, twice or even up to ten times in 24 hours (which can continue for weeks or months) are symptoms of cluster headaches. The pain then disappears in eight out of ten victims and goes into recess for months or years. It then comes back with its previous intensity for another devastating bout. The condition is often confused with trigeminal neuralgia because of the severity of the pain, but unlike trigeminal neuralgia, which strikes with stabs as brief as a lightning flash, the pains in cluster headache last from ten minutes to several hours at a time. It is also confused with migraine, hence the term "migrainous neuralgia," which is still preferred in Great Britain. But only in about 20 percent of all patients do the pains recur regularly, without intermission, in the manner of migraine.

Cluster headaches are thought to be an allergic reaction, since histamine is found in the tissue cells on the affected side. Histamine (a substance that causes capillaries and veins to dilate) is released when there is an injury to the skin or membranes, such as a reaction by the membranes to an allergen. Recent experimentation suggests lithium (a drug frequently used to treat manic depression) is a useful treatment for selected victims of cluster headache.

ICE-CREAM HEADACHES

Holding ice or ice cream in the mouth or swallowing it while it is still very cold may cause localized pain in the palate or throat. A headache in the forehead or temple because of referred pain from the trigeminal nerve endings may sometimes occur. Occasionally it may produce pain behind the ear because this area is supplied by another cranial nerve, the glossopharyngeal, which also has branches over the back of the throat that may be thrown into sudden activity by intense cold. The cause of ice-cream headache is sudden cooling of the roof of the mouth. Cooling of the esophagus (the tube which connects the throat with the stomach) or the stomach itself does not cause the pain. Obviously, the cure for ice-cream headache is either to avoid eating ice cream, or to ingest intensely cold substances at a slow and easy rate.

OTHER TYPES OF HEADACHES

Hypoglycemia

Hypoglycemia is a medical disorder in which the body's normal balance of blood sugar is impaired and, as a result, blood sugar levels drop. Hypoglycemia deprives the brain of needed glucose (sugar), and it is theorized that the physiological complications it triggers can lead to headaches. If you awake from a night's sleep with headaches (and it has probably been ten to twelve hours since you have eaten), you should consider the possibility that you may be experiencing hypoglycemia. The "Sunday morning headache" is fairly common among those who sleep late after a Saturday night of playing softball, dancing or other physical activity which lowers the blood sugar level. If you suspect that hypoglycemia may be a problem for you, consult your physician. Although hypoglycemia is probably less common than recent publicity suggests, it can usually be controlled with dietary modifications (Chapter 10).

Allergy Headaches

The exact association between headaches and allergy is not clear, but recent research does suggest that certain substances seem to act as triggering mechanisms. Of the substances most frequently mentioned, certain foods appear to be major culprits. There is now substantial research evidence linking foods that contain tyramine (beer, wine, cheese and most dairy products and some vegetables) with the onset of severe migraine-like headaches in susceptible individuals. Chocolate is also believed to trigger allergy headaches. The so-called "Chinese Restaurant Syndrome" headache is brought on by monosodium glutamate which is often used as a flavor-enhancer and is found in soy sauce. If you have headaches after eating hot dogs, bacon, ham or salami, you may be allergic to the nitrates used as coloring agents in these foods. See Chapter 10 for more about diet, allergy and headaches.

Sinus Headaches

A sinus headache is a symptom of nasal and sinus congestion and inflammation (sinusitis). It is characterized by a dull, throbbing ache around the eyes and cheekbones, which eventually spreads throughout the head. The nose is blocked on one or both sides, and the face often becomes "puffy" and tender. The sinuses are air pockets located in the bone of the forehead (frontal sinuses) and in the cheekbone on either side of the nose (maxillary sinuses); other air pockets are found behind the bridge of the nose (sphenoid and ethmoid sinuses). Air fills the sinuses whose secretions drain freely into the nose.

The sinuses play a major role in the normal resonance of the voice, which is why when we have a cold and the mucous membrane lining of the nose swells and blocks the small opening of the sinuses, our voices sound flat and lifeless without the usual timbre. It is thought that the mucous congestion in the nasal passages and sinus cavities impinges on neighboring nerves and blood vessels to initiate a sinus headache. The decreased amount of oxygen that is respired because of congestion may also cause the initiation of some compensatory measures, eventually resulting in a headache.

Chronic sinus headaches are not as prevalent as they are thought to be. They usually do not afflict sufferers of chronic sinus problems, but are often confused by these people and by many others with headaches caused by allergy, tension or other trigger factors that produce similar symptoms. If you think you are suffering from sinus headaches, you should consult a doctor.

Hangover Headaches

Alcohol is a potent dilator of blood vessels, and sufficient quantities of alcohol can trigger a severe headache. Excessive alcohol also can cause dehydration, depression of normal brain functioning, dissipation of vitamins B and C, and the addition of toxic irritants to the stomach. Add to that the excessive cigarette smoke, strenuous dancing and loud music which frequently accompany a "night on the town" and there is little wonder that participants wake the morning after with a headache.

Alcohol, however, was considered a medical phenomenon for centuries. Poets praised its restorative powers, claiming that they felt better, thought better and were closer to the gods under its influence. Physicians prescribed it as an aid for digestion, circulation, visibility, physical strength and even headaches. Since alcohol causes blood vessels to dilate, similar to the physiological change that occurs during vascular headaches, it is difficult to see how alcohol has any value in the treatment of headaches. Perhaps the beneficial effect of this prescription was psychological, the alcohol causing relaxation, altered consciousness or numbing of nerves to sufficiently raise the pain threshold. Nevertheless, today we know that a few ounces of alcohol will produce headaches in people who otherwise are seldom troubled with head pain.

Some alcoholic beverages are more toxic than others and cause worse hangovers. The so-called "hard" liquors such as brandy, bourbon, dark rum and rye usually produce the worst hangovers. Beverages such as scotch, blended whiskies, gin and vodka are generally thought to be less harsh to the body. However, the only sure way to prevent hangover headaches is to avoid drinking. For those who consume excessive amounts of alcohol two aspirins and a seltzer taken before going to bed may help. This may not totally eliminate the hangover, but it may make the morning after somewhat more bearable.

Brain Tumor Headaches

The one disorder that nearly every chronic headache sufferer wonders about at some time or another is brain tumor. Headaches are symptoms of some brain tumors, but not all of them. Only when the tumor enlarges sufficiently to press against a pain-sensitive structure does a headache result. Since much of the brain is insensitive to pain and much of it is not located in the area of a pain-sensitive structure, headaches are not a good indicator of brain tumor. In fact, only a very small percentage of headaches, perhaps less than one percent by some estimates, are caused by brain tumors. Symptoms more accurately suggestive of brain tumor include impairments in speech, vision and coordination, and personality changes.

A tumor is a collection of cells which multiply indiscriminately without the organization and control which characterize normal growth. A tumor is considered benign if it grows slowly, pushing other tissues aside, and restricts itself to one location. If the tumor grows rapidly and destroys normal tissue, it is termed malignant. Malignant tumors may separate and spread by way of lymph ducts or the bloodstream to other parts of the body. The malignant process in general is called cancer.

If your doctor believes that your headaches might possibly be the result of a brain tumor, he is likely to schedule you for extensive diagnostic testing. Testing may include X rays of the skull, tomography, isotope scanning, ultrasound, electroencephalogram (EEG) and a specialized battery of neuropsychological tests. Many brain tumors can be completely removed by a neurosurgeon with excellent results. With the steadily increasing sophistication of medical diagnosis and treatment, there are numerous alternatives available for the very small percentage of patients who suffer headache resulting from brain tumor. If the possibility of a brain tumor concerns you, contact your physician.

Eyestrain Headaches

Headaches resulting from eyestrain are usually associated with pain in and around the eye. They are occasionally confused with sinus headaches which cause pain in the maxillary sinus located just under the eyes. Eyestrain is caused by contraction of the muscles surrounding the eye, usually after prolonged use or because of impaired refraction. Writing, reading or other detailed work for long periods or in poor light can cause tension in the eye muscles as the eyes strain to focus properly and present clear images to the brain. A brief rest and simple proprietary drugs for pain usually relieve eyestrain headaches. If you experience headaches when reading, writing or doing detailed work, consult an ophthalmologist.

Glaucoma

Glaucoma, a disease caused by intense pressure in the eyeball, can also cause headaches. Other warning signs of glaucoma are the appearance of halos around lighted objects, blurred vision and depression. If untreated, glaucoma can lead to blindness; therefore, periodic testing for the disease by an ophthalmologist is recommended.

5

Medication for Headache Pain

Drugs are without question the most commonly used head-ache-relief method employed today. This is not without good reason: They are easy to administer and relatively inexpensive, and their effects are usually predictable. For a large number of headache sufferers, they work. It's hardly surprising that the vast pharmacopoeia of analegisic (pain-relieving) and prophylactic medication developed in the last twenty-five years have become the physician's first line of defense against headaches.

Unfortunately, medication is not effective for all headache sufferers; even when it is successful, it can still create problems. For example, drugs currently cure headaches that are of infectious origin only. Our available medication can often decrease the intensity of head pain, abort a headache attack in its early stage and, at times, prevent the onset of headache pain. However, there is currently no medication that effectively "cures" headaches. In fact, many of the more powerful drugs used to relieve headache distress can potentially cause serious side effects when used in large doses over an extended period of time. Serious psychological and physical dependence can also develop with certain medications. On occasion, physicians have watched in frustration as the patient's headaches and need for medication became two different responses: the headaches going their way, sometimes improving, sometimes becoming worse, and the addictive pattern taking a divergent course, always growing stronger.

PROPRIETARY ANALGESICS

Proprietary analgesics are also referred to as over-the-counter drugs since they can be purchased without a prescription. In general, you should not self-medicate without the advice of a physician if you:

1. have any other symptom associated with the headache
2. if headache is frequently recurrent or is a prolonged headache
3. have asthma or other allergic diseases or ulcers
4. have had past allergic reactions to aspirin or other pain medications
5. take medication which affects blood clotting
6. have a history of gout, arthritis or diabetes.

The above conditions represent instances where medications may have adverse effects on underlying disorders. In addition, the presence of any of the above factors should strongly encourage you to consult your physician.

Aspirin

Aspirin (acetylsalicylic acid) is a highly effective and important member of those analgesics classified as nonnarcotics and, moreover, is the single most widely used drug in the world—narcotic and nonnarcotic alike (Table 5-1). In addition to its use as an analgesic, aspirin also has antipyretic (reduces fever) and anti-inflammation (reduces noninfectious redness and swelling) properties. Because aspirin is a nonprescription drug and so readily available, it is generally not always credited with the analgesic efficacy it in fact possesses. When compared to other analgesics, aspirin is effective, useful, inexpensive and has a relatively low incidence of adverse side effects.

Aspirin and other nonnarcotic analgesics appear to reduce

pain by interfering with the biochemistry of pain formation at peripheral nerve sites in the body. Unlike narcotic analgesics, aspirin does not alter the response to pain in the central nervous system, and therefore has a lower analgesic effect. For example, 650 mgs of aspirin is generally thought to produce as much pain relief as 60 mgs of codeine.* Doses of aspirin exceeding 650 mgs, however, do not increase peak analgesia (although the duration of effect may be prolonged), whereas increased doses of codeine, for instance, will provide greater relief from pain. Aspirin, it seems, has a "ceiling effect" around 650 mgs, and doses beyond that amount do little to increase its effectiveness. Aspirin may have some slight effects on central nervous system activity, but compared to the effects of morphine and other narcotic analgesics, the effects of aspirin are negligible.

Although aspirin is relatively safe, does not cause physical dependence and is readily available, it can produce side effects, such as heartburn, nausea, gastric irritation and possibly gastric bleeding. Aspirin also reduces the tendency of blood to clot, thereby prolonging bleeding time. Significant overmedication can cause aspirin toxicity which could possibly be fatal. The symptoms of extreme aspirin poisoning include hypothermia (loss of body heat), cardiac arrhythmia (irregular heart beat), shallow breathing, coma and death. When treated properly, however, most cases of aspirin poisoning are not life-threatening. Ringing of ears or dizziness may signal approaching toxicity; if you experience either condition, see your physician.

Acetaminophen

Acetaminophen (Datril®, Tylenol®, Liquiprin® and others)

*A combination of 650 mgs of aspirin and 32 mgs of codeine is stronger than 60 mgs of codeine (taken orally) and 32 mgs of Darvon®; it is as strong as or equal to 650 mgs of acetaminophen and 65 mgs of Darvon®.

is approximately equal in analgesic strength to aspirin and has a mode of action in the body that is also similar to aspirin (Table 5-1). Acetaminophen has enjoyed a surge of popularity in recent years as an effective analgesic that does not cause the minor gastric irritation and bleeding that can result from aspirin intake.

Acetaminophen is both an analgesic and antipyretic. The analgesic effect is achieved with one (325 mg) or two tablets. Taking more tablets is both useless and perhaps dangerous, depending on the quantity and the individual. In excessive doses, acetaminophen can cause fatal liver damage (excessive in this case can be as few as thirty tablets, although death rarely occurs with fewer than forty tablets). As mentioned, aspirin can also be fatally abused, but it is a much slower-acting analgesic. Overdoses of aspirin follow a progressive pattern into coma and shock. For muscle-contraction headache victims acetaminophen can be an effective medication.

TABLE 5-1

PROPRIETARY ANALGESICS

Plain Aspirin Tablets

Most aspirin tablets are somewhat similarly manufactured and differ primarily in price. However, there are a few products that are less well manufactured and can be either too hard or too soft. Tightly compressed tablets do not readily dissolve, while loose crumbled tablets can contain degraded drugs. These products often have a vinegar odor and should not be taken since they have pharmaceutical differences which can be clinically important.

Buffered Aspirin

The buffering process theoretically offers some advantage due to the frequent stomach irritation of unbuffered aspirin. However, this product is usually more expensive than plain aspirin.

Buffered Aspirin Solutions

Although these solutions (usually liquid) can give rapid and effective relief, they generally increase urinary excretion of salicylate. The large sodium content and decrease in salicylate blood levels make these products unsuitable for long-term administration but very effective for occasional treatment of headache.

Combinations

Generally not as suitable for long-term administration but appropriate for occasional treatment of headache. A major problem is the large sodium content in this type of medication.

Time-Released Aspirin

No significant advantage has been consistently determined.

Enteric-Coated Aspirin

These tablets are coated with a substance that does not dissolve until reaching the intestine, where the drug is then released. Since it takes longer to produce pain relief, this type of medication is not generally used for treatment of headaches, though it is most appropriate for patients with a history of ulcers or severe gastric distress.

Aspirin Combinations

Some aspirin combinations contain phenacetin and/or caffeine and may be less effective than other available preparations. In addition, aspirin combinations are thought to produce more adverse side effects and generally are not considered most appropriate for treatment of headache.

*Information for the patient taking aspirin:
Aspirin tablets should be taken with eight ounces of water after meals or, if appropriate, with an antacid. All aspirin should be kept in a tightly closed bottle in a cool dry place and out of the reach of children. The bathroom is not a good place for storing aspirin because of dampness. Throw away any aspirin that smells like vinegar.

Acetaminophen
Frequently a drug of choice for mild to moderate headache, acetaminophen produces less stomach irritation than aspirin and is less likely to cause allergic reactions. For patients who are aspirin-intolerant, take oral anticoagulants or have a history of peptic ulcer disease or asthma, acetaminophen is also a useful and effective drug.

*Information for the patient taking acetaminophen:
Be careful not to exceed the specified dosage and dosing intervals for this medication. Ten to 60 minutes is usually required for this drug to be effective and the effects will normally last from six to eight hours. Do not take acetaminophen regularly for more than 10 days without consulting your physician.

Extra-Strength Pain Relievers
There are generally two types of extra-strength proprietary analgesics. The first type combines more than one analgesic into a single product, and the total ingredient of aspirin usually exceeds 325 mgs. The second type usually contains more than 325 mgs of the same drug.

Often one "extra-strength" preparation is nearly equal to two capsules or tablets of regular strength; therefore it is often implied that "extra-strength" drugs are more effective, although results vary. The primary advantage of this type of medication may be that the patient must swallow fewer capsules or tablets.

PRESCRIPTION ANALGESICS

Prescription analgesics must be prescribed by a physician. Since there are a number of prescription analgesics available, we will review several popular prescription analgesics frequently used for head pain.

Codeine

Codeine preparations are effective in reducing pain, but may cause drowsiness and/or sedation. For this reason, patients should be very careful when performing activities which require alertness or fast reaction time, such as driving an automobile. In addition, care should be exercised to insure that other drugs which cause drowsiness are not taken with codeine since the additive effect is potentially dangerous. Codeine may be habit-forming.

Nonsteroidal Anti-Inflammatory Agents

These medications, which include Motrin®, Naprosyn®, Anaprox® and Zomax®, were primarily designed for certain forms of arthritis but have been shown to have significant pain-relief potential as well. Though these drugs are being increasingly used for pain relief, specific prescribing of these drugs for headaches remains a broad practice and is still in the process of being fully evaluated by the U.S. Federal Drug Administration. These drugs should be taken with milk or food. They may cause nausea, vomiting or heartburn, as well as possible allergic reactions. Dizziness, blurring of vision and easy bruising should be reported to your physician.

Pentazosine

Pentazosine (Talwin®) has been proven to be a moderately effective pain reliever for mild to moderate pain, but it can also cause drowsiness and/or sedation. Care should therefore be taken when one drives or participates in activities requiring alertness. Also, mood changes and hallucinations have been reported with the use of Talwin®. This medication may be habit-forming.

Propoxyphene

Propoxyphene (Darvon®) has been used extensively in recent years for relief of headache pain, although a number of potential side effects have been reported. Darvon® may cause drowsiness, dizziness or nausea and should *not* be taken with alcoholic beverages. It is for the above reasons that Darvon® is currently less frequently used than in the past.

Butalbital/Aspirin/Phenacetin/Caffeine

This combination of medications (Fiorinal®) is frequently prescribed for mild to moderate muscle-contraction headaches. It may cause drowsiness and may adversely interact with a number of other medications. Gastric distress is a particularly common problem. In addition, there is concern that this medication may be habit-forming when used for a prolonged period of time.

ERGOTAMINE TARTRATE

The most widely used antimigraine drug is ergotamine

tartrate, a vasoconstrictor and derivative of the fungus *Claviceps purpura*, which grows on damp and mouldy grains. Ergotamine tartrate is contained in many drugs prescribed for migraine headaches, but it is not classified an analgesic. This ingredient constricts the cranial arteries, thereby preventing the migraine attack from developing. Ergotamine was first introduced in the United States in 1934 and has been proven clinically effective in aborting an oncoming migraine attack in as high as 70 percent of the patients studied. Its advantages are threefold:

1. It is not a hypnotic drug and has only minimal effect on the mental or emotional processes of most patients.
2. It works quickly to terminate a migraine attack and is more effective than any other currently available chemical remedy.
3. It usually relieves a number of symptoms associated with migraine, as well as the headache.

Because ergotamine works to abort the onset of migraine and does not relieve pain, the drug dosage must be individualized and taken *before* the arteries become too dilated. Patients must carry the drug with them at all times in order to have it available at the very first sign of an oncoming headache. After the drug is taken, you should retire to a quiet, dimly-lit room and go to sleep. If a migraine victim makes the mistake of taking ergotamine and continuing with planned activities, headache relief will be temporary, the headache often returning with renewed force. The use of ergotamine tartrate, then, should follow this five-stage pattern:

1. Realization of a pending migraine attack.
2. Immediate cessation of activities.
3. Dosage of ergotamine tartrate, administered by, or with the consent of a physician. (*Do not exceed prescribed dosage!*)

4. Rest and sleep.
5. Modified schedule for at least one day following the onset of headache.

Ergotamine tartrate is an effective interventive drug for many migraine headache sufferers, but a number of contraindications and serious side effects associated with chronic usage can result. One possible complication is dependency on ergotamine with daily use. Increased tolerance may result in increased frequency of headaches which follow withdrawal of the drug. Continued heavy use of ergotamine seems to have an effect on the central nervous system which could contribute to emotional disturbances. In addition, another major potential adverse effect is ergotism, a condition that occurs when the capillaries in the arms and legs become so constricted that they cannot conduct blood to the tips of the fingers and toes. With circulation completely cut off, victims experience severe burning sensations in their extremities. Thanks to modern pharmacological control, ergotism is extremely rare today.

Occasional physiological side effects of ergotamine tartrate include nausea, vomiting, gastric discomfort, diarrhea, parethesias (numbness or tingling) of the extremities, stiffness of the thigh and neck muscles, generalized weakness, transient tachycardia (abnormal rapidity of heartbeat) and localized edema (swelling) and itching in sensitive patients. Ergotamine tartrate drugs should be taken with food, and the prescribed dosage *should not* be exceeded. Table 5-2 lists by brand name a number of drugs containing ergotamine tartrate.

ERGOTAMINE TARTRATE COMBINATION

Since some types of headaches are thought to be caused by dilated cranial blood vessels, it is not surprising that other chemicals known to act as vasoconstrictors have been used in attempts to prevent headache. The combination of ergotamine tartrate and caffeine is today frequently prescribed as a prophylactic agent. In fact, coffee is considered by some headache experts to be therapeutic in this instance since the caffeine in coffee acts as a vasoconstrictor and accelerates the effect of ergotamine. The combination of ergotamine and caffeine is packaged in three ways: in sublingual form (to be placed under the tongue until dissolved), in pill form (to be chewed at the first sign of a migraine attack) and in suppository form. Chewing pills facilitates rapid absorption in the body, while suppositories insure absorption in those victims who frequently vomit during migraine attacks.

When consumed in coffee, caffeine can liberate glucose for quick use in the brain. The release of glucose may help speed recovery from nutritional headaches (Chapter 10). This does not mean that twenty cups of coffee a day will prevent a migraine attack; the deleterious effects of so much caffeine are well known. Nevertheless, in theory at least, coffee and medications containing caffeine, when taken in proper amounts at strategic times in association with ergotamine, can be helpful in aborting a migraine attack. Table 5-2 lists examples of drugs by brand name that contain combinations of ergotamine tartrate and caffeine.

OTHER PROPHYLACTIC MEDICATIONS

There are a number of other medications of proven value that can reduce the frequency of migraine attacks when taken two or three times a day as a preventive measure. First among these are agents that block the direct effects of serotonin on the blood vessels, where it could be responsible for constriction of small arteries and for sensitizing vessels to cause pain. Serotonin is in many ways a mystery substance whose actions and reactions are demonstrable but not fully revealed. It is found in greatest amounts in the midbrain and hypothalamus, parts of the brain which regulate the body's reaction to stress situations. It is thought to affect the emotional states by its presence or absence in these regions. The psychedelic drug lysergic acid diethylamide (LSD) is similar in composition to serotonin. In fact, LSD was accidentally synthesized by a chemist looking for a serotonin-inhibiting substance to treat migraines.

TABLE 5-2

SOME MEDICATIONS FREQUENTLY PRESCRIBED FOR HEADACHE*

Proprietary Drugs

Analgesics

Bufferin	Aspirin	Tylenol	Vanquish
Excedrin	Datril	Liquiprin	Cope

Prescription Drugs

Analgesics	Interventive (vasoconstrictors)		Prophylactic
Codeine	(Ergotamine	(Ergotamine	Sansert
Fiorinal	Tartrate)	Combinations)	Inderal
	Gynergen	Cafergot	
	Ergomar	Cafergot PB	
		Migral	

*The following drugs, with the exception of aspirin, are registered trademarks. Their listing here is for reader's information and not an endorsement.

TABLE 5-2

SOME MEDICATIONS FREQUENTLY PRESCRIBED FOR HEADACHE *continued*

Psychotropic Drugs

Antianxiety Drugs

Minor Tranquillizers*		Phenothiazines	
Valium	Librium	Thorazine	Prolixin
Serax	Ativan	Trilifon	Stelazine
Vistaril	Tranxene	Mellaril	Serentil

Antidepressant Drugs

Tricyclic		MAO inhibitor	
Norpramine	Sinequan	Parnate	Nardil
Elavil	Vivactin	Marplan	Marsilid
Tofranil	Surmontil		

Methysergide (Sansert®) is one of the most effective serotonin-inhibiting prophylactic agents for migraine. However, it is not used for the *acute* migraine attack. Its main disadvantage is that about one in three patients who take it for the first time experience aching of the arms or legs, gastrointestinal distress or other unusual symptoms for several days afterward. While these symptoms usually disappear, 10 percent of the patients who take this drug are not able to tolerate it. Of the other 90 percent, many either experience a cessation of headaches or suffer less than half the previous frequency. Because of its chemical similarity to ergotamine, it is not recommended for pregnant women or for people

---

*The terms major and minor when applied to tranquillizers do not refer to the drug's physiological effects; the terms refer to the chemical structure and action of the tranquillizer.

suffering from liver, kidney or vascular disease or any form of gastrointestinal disorder.

Methysergide should be taken daily with food, but its use should be stopped altogether for one month in every four to prevent the development of fibrous tissues, a major adverse reaction. Methysergide may cause drowsiness, and persons taking it should avoid abrupt postural change. If extremities cramp or become numb or cold, call your physician. Because of these potential problems, this medication is used selectively.

Propanolol hydrochloride (Inderal®) is another medication that has enjoyed a recent popularity in the prophylaxis of migraine headaches. It is more commonly known for its use in the treatment of hypertension (high blood pressure), but it has recently been demonstrated to be frequently effective in the prevention of the onset of vascular headaches. The mechanism of the antimigraine effect of Inderal has not been established, but some speculate that this drug prevents arterial spasms when taken on a daily basis. The patient most likely to benefit from Inderal is one who has experienced migraine headaches of long duration and has had pulsating or throbbing pain on one side of the head accompanied by nausea, vomiting and sensitivity to light.

If no satisfactory response to Inderal treatment is obtained in four to six weeks, its use is usually discontinued. On withdrawal, it is usually advisable to reduce the dosage gradually over several weeks to avoid possible cardiac complications. Among the major disadvantages of Propanolol is fatigue and occasional insomnia.

PSYCHOTROPIC MEDICATIONS

Doctors and researchers have long implicated psychological variables in the etiology of headaches. Much has been said in health-care circles about the migraine personality and the role of anxiety and depression in both migraine and muscle-contraction headaches. The existence of a true migraine personality is questionable, and the role of psychological variables in pain is not fully understood.

Clinically, however, it is generally accepted that many chronic-headache sufferers also experience psychological problems (such as anxiety and depression) which must be considered when formulating a treatment plan. Whether anxiety and depression precipitate headaches or vice versa is debatable. Nevertheless, pharmacological therapy for headaches often involves the administration of antianxiety and antidepressant medication.

Antianxiety Drugs

One of the variables that must be taken into account when a physician prescribes a drug for pain, including headaches, is to what extent the patient's anxiety may be causing or intensifying the pain. Muscle-contraction headaches resulting from tension or stress are the most likely to respond to antianxiety drugs, although some migraine victims report a decrease in headache frequency and intensity.

Phenothiazines and benzodiazepines are the two chemical classes most often used to control anxiety. Phenothiazines have a number of side effects, but low dosages of this type of drug may possibly produce less severe side effects than associated with benzodiazepine drugs. For example, a physician may prescribe a benzodiazepine (Valium®, Librium®) for muscle relaxation and/or anxiety for a patient suffering from muscle-contraction headaches. Some patients may become depressed as a result of long-term Valium use. While Valium may effectively reduce the suffering of anxiety and muscle-contraction headaches, it may also reduce the body's ability to tolerate pain, cause depression and/or drug dependence, and may interfere with natural sleep patterns. Short-term use is therefore preferable, especially since dependency is a potential problem.

The phenothiazine tranquillizers appear to be effective in reducing the frequency of many tension-headache patterns and, in the long term, may possibly have less potential for causing depression. They are effective because they block receptor sites for two chemicals in the brain, dopamine and norepinephrine, which are thought to increase pain tolerance. In addition, phenothiazines also assist in the control of anxiety when administered in small doses. However, they have significant potential side effects, such as restlessness and abnormal body jerking, and should be used with caution and under careful supervision, particularly if used on a long-term basis.

Antidepressant Drugs

The use of antidepressant medication for recurrent headaches is a relatively new, but promising application of these drugs. There are basically three types of antidepressant medications available: tricyclic antidepressants, monoamine oxidase inhibitors and psychostimulants. The latter group is seldom recommended for headache relief.

The tricyclic antidepressants help to relieve depression by increasing the supply of certain neurosynaptic transmitter chemicals (norepinephrine, serotonin and dopamine) in the brain. However, not all tricyclic antidepressants have the same effect since they may involve norepinephrine, serotonin and dopamine alone or in some combination. As a rule, the tricyclic antidepressants take from four to fourteen days to achieve maintenance levels, and the maximum effective response therefore often does not occur for two to four weeks after treatment has begun. Most tricyclic drugs have similar potential side effects, including dryness of the mouth, excessive sweating, transient vision problems (blurring), constipation and urinary retention. More serious are the potential cardiovascular effects which preclude use by many patients, particularly those with preexisting cardiovascular disease. In view of all possible side effects, tricyclic antidepressants must be used most cautiously in patients with hypertension, glaucoma, prostatism (any condition with obstruction of the prostate gland), chronic heart disease and epilepsy.

Some patients who have not responded favorably to tricyclic antidepressants have very infrequently been given a trial on monoamine oxidase (MAO) inhibitors. These chemicals work as antidepressants; they increase the concentration of available neurotransmitters by inhibiting their metabolism by monoamine oxidase. If neurotransmitters are not metabolized, there will be more of them. A greater supply should have an effect on depression caused by a deficiency of neurotransmitters in the brain.

MAO inhibitors have a number of serious side effects and should be used only in severe cases where tricyclic antidepressants have failed. Patients taking MAO inhibitors must be extremely careful to avoid any food containing tyramine, since those foods may interact to cause a rapid elevation of blood pressure and severe headache, nausea, vomiting and sometimes fatal cerebral hemorrhage. Foods rich in tyramine include wine, cheese, anchovies, pickles, yogurt, snails and chicken liver.

Stimulant drugs such as amphetamines were used by some physicians in the treatment of depression because of their rapid effect of increasing physical and mental activity. However, because of their questionable effectiveness, particularly in pain states such as headaches, they are seldom used today. The disadvantage of stimulant drugs are many: They cause anorexia (loss of appetite), habituation such that more and more of the drug is needed to produce an effect, addiction, jitteriness, and can result in a toxic amphetamine psychosis. The use of stimulant drugs in the treatment of headaches is therefore *not* recommended.

SPECIAL CONSIDERATION FOR THE ELDERLY

In general, drug dosages for elderly patients should be reduced from average adult levels, and the frequency of administration should be decreased. This recommendation is made because of varying general responses in elderly patients, as well as varying excretion rates. The best rule to follow is to start slowly and proceed slowly. This rule may help avoid overmedication and resulting dizziness and imbalance.

DRUG-INDUCED HEADACHES

Some drugs produce headaches as a common and expected side effect. Examples are isosorbide dinitrate (Isordil®), nitroglycerin and oral contraceptives. In the case of isosorbide and nitroglycerin, this side effect is common and expected and suggests that the medication remains effective. However, if you have headaches with oral contraceptives, your physician should be consulted.

IN CONCLUSION

The analgesic you choose over-the-counter or the drug your physician prescribes to treat your headache should involve both patient-specific and drug factors. Past history of asthma. hypersensitivity reactions, stomach problems and problems with other medications will be very important in choosing the right drug for you.

6

Surgery for
Headache Relief

Surgery is today considered to be a last resort for that extremely small percentage of vascular headache sufferers who find themselves nearly totally incapacitated due to constant and severe head pain. Surgical treatment for headache relief is greatly influenced by what is known as the *specificity theory* of pain, which postulates that pain messages travel along "superhighway" nerve pathways in the body from the point of pain origin to the brain. The brain then analyzes and interprets the pain message and directs the body to react in some way. For example, accidentally placing a hand on the burner of a hot stove triggers the transmission of messages up nerve pathways to the brain. The brain receives the messages, interprets them as pain, and directs us to jerk our hand away from the painful stimulus—all in a fraction of a second. Removing the hand may avoid further tissue damage, but the injured area sends a continuous series of messages which the brain interprets as a steady throbbing pain in the hand. Surgery for pain relief is based on the logical assumption that if the pain pathway is interrupted, pain messages will not reach the brain and pain will not be experienced.

There are a number of disorders where surgery for relief of pain can be valuable and highly effective. In most cases where surgery is performed, pain results from some peripheral organic disorder such as a tumorous malignancy or scarring of the peripheral nerves from an injury. For specific types of painful disorders, such as trigeminal neuralgia (a type of facial pain which follows the distribution of the trigeminal nerve), surgery can often provide welcome relief.

Unfortunately, most disorders which result in constant or recurrent pain are fairly diffuse. Identification of a specific pain pathway is difficult, if not impossible. In addition, pain messages are continuously analyzed and interpreted all along the central nervous system, making isolation of a specific point for surgical interruption of pain pathways a complex task. In the case of severe headaches—one type of pain whose sources and pathways of transmission can be extremely difficult to isolate—there is little doubt in the medical field that surgery does not yet have the scientifically documented efficacy required of such a drastic treatment technique.

SURGERY FOR NONHEADACHE PAIN

Surgery for nonheadache pain has been performed at numerous body sites, from the remote peripheral nerves to the brain itself. The three most common sites are at the periphery, close to the pain site; at a limited number of locations along the spinal cord; and within selected areas of the brain.

Surgery at a peripheral site is called a neurectomy. This surgery may be performed on certain nerves in the leg to stop the transmission of pain messages from a damaged foot. Neurectomy is also sometimes performed on the trigeminal nerve to separate the nerve from nearby blood vessels which may be crowding and pressing on the nerve and causing severe pain in the cheek and face.

Three common types of surgery performed in the area of the spinal cord are rhizotomy, cordotomy and sympathectomy. These surgeries involve severing or cauterizing by electrical current nerves or nerve pathways. Rhizotomies are usually performed for pain in limited areas such as low-back pain; cordotomies for more diffuse, widespread pain. Sympathectomies are performed for a variety of pain disorders, including vascular headaches.

In many cases, these surgical procedures do not give permanent relief from pain. In fact, in most cases these procedures tend to lose their effectiveness in one to five years. Many authorities believe that pain recurs because severed or cauterized nerves regenerate and once again open the highway on which pain messages travel. Other researchers believe that adjacent nerves left intact during surgery gradually adapt and serve as secondary roads for transmission of pain messages. Occasionally, surgery causes scarring of nerve fibres, which can also cause pain.

In extremely severe cases, surgical procedures have been performed directly on the brain. These surgeries are rarely performed and are not intended to interrupt the transmission of pain messages. Surgeries such as prefrontal lobotomy, thalamotomy, mesencephalic tractomy and gyrectomy attempt to alter the response to pain sensations, much in the same way that morphine is used to alleviate suffering. When successful, brain surgery produces an effect comparable to that of morphine: The pain sensations are usually undiminished and the patient's pain threshold may be unchanged, but the pain is perceived as void of those negative qualities that make pain the objectionable perception that it usually is. Like other surgical procedures noted, brain surgery may also lose its pain-relief effectiveness in time and also has a high risk of affecting other aspects of the patient's behavior.

SURGERY FOR HEAD PAIN

Surgery for relief of headaches should be considered only in the most extremely severe cases and only after all other treatments have failed to bring relief. In addition to the concerns associated with general anesthesia and surgery in general, surgery for headache relief has a variable history of long-term positive results.

The surgical treatment of headaches has consisted primarily of procedures performed at three levels: vascular, sympathetic, and afferent sensory pathway.

Vascular

Early surgical intervention at the vascular level had consisted primarily of ligation (tying or binding) of various branches of the common carotid artery. The right and left common carotid arteries, both of which arise from the aorta (main trunk of the arterial system of the body arising from the upper surface of the left ventricle of the heart) are the principal blood suppliers to the head. Ligation of the common carotid was performed to reduce distention of the vessel walls which were assumed to be involved in headache. However, the therapeutic value of this technique has been increasingly questioned, and the procedure is very rarely performed today.

Sympathetic

The therapeutic rationale for sympathectomies is based upon the observation that the procedure appears to prevent vasospasm. The inhibition of vascular spasm is believed to be potentially useful in aborting the development of secondary chemical changes which follow initial vasospasms, resulting in the onset of painful vascular dilation. Sympathectomy involves excising a portion of a nerve of the sympathetic division of the autonomic nervous system. In twelve cases treated by unilateral sympathectomy at Middlesex Hospital in London, one researcher recently reported that three patients experienced complete relief of headaches, seven reported decreases in severity and frequency of attacks and two patients reported no change in headache activity.

Afferent Sensory Pathway

Sectioning of the involved afferent (incoming towards the brain) sensory pathways is a technique designed to block transmission of pain messages originating from an affected peripheral site. The afferent pathways primarily implicated in this approach are the superficial branches of the trigeminal nerve. Many neurosurgeons recommend sensory root sectioning only when the pain is repeated and severe, and the use of ergotamine drugs (Chapter 5) causes complications. Other doctors are quick to emphasize the potential dangers involved in such serious surgical intervention, which, in most cases, preclude its use. There has been some recent research indicating that pain tends to reappear after several months of diminution following surgery to sever pain pathways.

Cryosurgery

A more recent approach to the surgical treatment of vascular headaches is cryosurgery. This procedure generally involves the freezing of occipital, superficial temporal and spheno-palatine arteries (arteries located in the head) in a single operation. While the rationale for the effectiveness of this procedure is uncertain, some researchers believe that portions of these arteries are susceptible to extreme cold, and the procedure therefore selectively destroys these portions while the arteries stay intact. In a six-month follow-up study done in Great Britain in which 96 patients responded to a questionnaire, 41 reported a 75 percent or better improvement, while 12 patients reported elimination of their headaches. The status of the remaining 43 patients was not indicated.

SUMMARY

The effects of various types of surgery for headache relief are not convincing when considered in relation to less intrusive treatment alternatives. Exceptions, of course, are for the removal of tumors and, less frequently, nerve blocks. Adverse side effects of surgery for pain relief include numbness, loss of temperature sensitivity and the transference of the original pain site to a different part of the body. All things considered, surgery for headaches should be considered only in the most extremely severe cases and after all possible alternative treatments have been exhausted.

7

Biofeedback

The term biofeedback has come into popular usage in recent years in both scientific and popular circles. While still in its infancy, a considerable body of scientific research is fast developing which serves to clarify the role of biofeedback in the treatment of chronic pain [including migraine and muscle-contraction headaches.] First, biofeedback is not a product of our contemporary scientific age but is as old as mankind. Second, biofeedback is not a miracle cure, and it will not revolutionize health care. It will not cure cancer, leukemia, heart disease or the common cold! Biofeedback is simply a treatment technique—a proven, effective treatment technique in carefully selected patients suffering a limited number of medical disorders which have not consistently responded well to traditional medical practices. It is not a "cure-all," but is just one technique in a practitioner's armamentarium.

To understand biofeedback, a careful distinction must first be made between the terms "biofeedback" and "biofeedback training." Biofeedback is a natural, usually unconscious learning process. For example, how did you learn the complex mind—body coordination required to pick up a pencil, to write your name, to walk, to feed yourself without making

NOTE: This chapter is excerpted from *Managing Chronic Pain: A Patient's Guide*, pp. 63–74.

a mess, to throw a baseball, to play golf or to drive a car? The answer is biofeedback. Through trial-and-error efforts we receive feedback from the environment and our body which we then use to modify and perfect future efforts. For instance, the proper swing of a golf club requires the complex coordination of our muscles, nervous system and sensory systems of sight and touch. Through repeated trial-and-error feedback we refine and improve our coordination and are eventually rewarded with a lower golf score. Slightly more sophisticated types of biofeedback include listening to your heart rate with a stethoscope, weighing yourself on a bathroom scale, taking your blood pressure and taking your temperature with a thermometer. Biofeedback, then, is the measuring or recording of a biological process which is fed back (or made available) to the individual.

If an individual takes a biological process which is measured in some way and continuously "fed back" to him, and he attempts to use the information to guide his trial-and-error efforts to modify a targeted biological process, he is using biofeedback training. For instance, suppose you wanted to learn to decrease your heart rate. You might sit in a chair with a stethoscope to your chest and, through trial and error, attempt different mental strategies until you audibly detected a noticeable decrease. While this is a crude and simplistic example of biofeedback training, it does qualify under our definition. However, if your doctor refers you to a biofeedback specialist for training, don't expect your treatment to be this elementary.

Today biofeedback training for selected medical disorders refers to a variety of techniques utilizing sensitive and highly sophisticated biological recording instruments. To look at a fully equipped biofeedback facility is to be reminded of endless stereo components stacked one on the other with meters, dials and flashing lights. These instruments assist individuals in gaining conscious control over biological processes generally thought not to be under voluntary control. Through electronic measurement, integration, amplification and transformation into easily perceived visual and audio signals, one can sit passively and watch one's blood pressure vary from moment to moment or observe the electrical activity of painful muscles in the neck and back. Combined with other proven effective treatment techniques, biofeedback training is a useful component in the treatment of chronic pain.

Historical Perspective

Scientists and laymen alike have long been fascinated with Far East yogis who reportedly can walk on broken glass and survive extended periods of time submerged under water without oxygen. The ability to achieve such voluntary control of physiological mechanisms has remained a mystery until about twenty years ago when science began its first serious look at meditation and associated forms of mind-body interactions. Experimentation first began with laboratory animals, but as research and understanding grew, the use of human subjects became commonplace. Let's look at some of the historical highlights in the development of biofeedback from an early mystic phenomenon to an accepted and effective treatment technique.

The roots of the scientific study of biofeedback training can be traced back to the 1960's when Dr. Neil Miller, a psychologist, and his colleagues reported they had successfully trained a number of laboratory rats to voluntarily control their heart rates, blood pressures and formation of urine. Dr. Miller, in fact, claimed that the rats could even be trained to increase the blood flow to one ear while maintaining the natural flow of blood to the other! Needless to say, this report sparked the interest of the scientific community, and the scientifically controlled experimentation of biofeedback began.

Early reports of laboratory animals taught to raise and lower blood pressure, alter blood flow, and increase and decrease their heart rates also met with much skepticism. Biofeedback was in direct contradiction to what had long been accepted as scientific fact: that our bodily processes are controlled by either the voluntary nervous system (e.g., arm and leg movements) or the involuntary nervous system (e.g., heart rate, digestion, blood pressure, etc.). It is true that our hearts will beat without our conscious efforts and that our blood pressure will vary from moment to moment "automatically." However, early biofeedback research demonstrated that we can learn to exert some conscious control over biological processes previously assumed to be totally beyond our control. This was considered a major scientific breakthrough, and the number of researchers investigating biofeedback grew rapidly.

Some twenty years after the beginning of serious scientific investigation of biofeedback, we find that the treatment modality is no longer only speculative laboratory research, but a proven clinical treatment technique. Once a counterculture fad with interest targeted toward achieving nirvana and inner peace through alpha wave feedback, biofeedback training is today performed by thousands of doctors and therapists in treating a variety of chronic-pain conditions such as migraine headaches, tension headaches, low-back pain, Raynaud's disease and temporomandibular joint pain. Biofeedback training has come of age and has gained wide acceptance. . . .

Biofeedback Training: Technique

The most effective use of biofeedback training in the treatment of chronic-pain conditions has focussed on learning voluntary control of one of the following physiological processes: electromyographic biofeedback and thermal biofeedback. Electromyographic (more commonly referred to as EMG) biofeedback is most frequently employed in the treatment of musculoskeletal disorders. Electrical activity of targeted muscle groups is recorded and made continuously available to patients who use this information, along with instructions from the therapist, to gradually learn better control of "tight" or "tense" muscles.

A second frequently employed type of biofeedback in the treatment of chronic pain is known as thermal or temperature biofeedback. Thermal biofeedback is most often the treatment of choice with vascular disorders involving impaired blood circulation in the body, usually the head, hands or feet. Blood flow from an affected body part is recorded and made continuously available to patients who combine the knowledge with instructions from the therapist to increase or decrease circulation to the [head].

Most patients who undergo biofeedback training are referred by their physician to a biofeedback therapist or doctor who uses biofeedback as one of several techniques in the treatment of [head pain].* If you are referred for biofeedback training, you should remember that biofeedback treatment is much different than other forms of health care to which you may be accustomed. In biofeedback training, the patient must assume responsibility for his health care and expend the effort required to learn and effectively utilize biofeedback skills. Of course, the doctor or therapist will assist you in your

---

*Unfortunately, neither the Federal Drug Administration nor state governments have yet passed legislation restricting the purchase of biofeedback instruments and the practice of biofeedback training to physicians, clinical psychologists and dentists. As a result, biofeedback techniques are being used by educators, counselors and a host of weakly certified or noncertified medical and psychological therapists. Before treatment, ensure that the practitioner holds a doctorate in medicine, clinical psychology or dentistry.

training, but the final responsibility falls on the patient. The doctor or therapist acts much like a coach, teaching and directing you as you learn a new skill to combat chronic pain. This approach is in sharp contrast to traditional health care where the doctor assumes responsibility for our health care. Rather than handing you pills to take for your pain, the biofeedback therapist will help you learn ways to manage your pain.

Should you decide that biofeedback is worth a trial, you will learn that biofeedback training involves several phases. The order of the phases and the specifics of treatment will vary with the doctor or therapist and the type of [headaches] you have. However, the following protocol should give you some idea of what to expect from biofeedback training.

The first phase of biofeedback training is termed the baseline phase. After your doctor or biofeedback therapist conducts a careful evaluation of your pain and before feedback training begins, you may be asked to keep a "pain diary" for a week or two. Careful daily charting of your pain intensity and the name and amount of any medication taken will give your doctor or therapist valuable information. For example, in addition to obtaining a baseline measure of your pain intensity and medication intake (which can be used for comparison as you progress in biofeedback training), important pain patterns or trends can often be identified. Baseline measurement prior to beginning biofeedback training is an attempt to provide a degree of control and objectivity to your self-reported pain complaints. It is to the patient's benefit to cooperate and carefully complete the Daily Pain Diary as requested.

Once a baseline has been established, your doctor or therapist will orient you to the biofeedback equipment. You will likely be requested to sit in a comfortable chair, usually located in a dimly lit, sound-resistant room. Your doctor or therapist will explain the operation of the biofeedback equipment, which looks like a collection of stereo components complete with meters, lights and calibration gauges. Depending on where you are experiencing your pain, the skin around the affected body part will be cleaned with alcohol or acetone. This will cleanse the skin of oil and promote the best contact between your skin and the electrodes.

The electrodes (which measure muscle activity or blood flow, depending on the type of biofeedback employed) are next secured to the skin with an adhesive collar. The placement of the electrodes is often directly on the painful body part. Two or three electrodes may be used, with one electrode serving as a ground. You will then be asked to relax while the biofeedback equipment is calibrated and checked.

The next step involves measuring the normal or resting level of the biological process targeted for training. For instance, if your pain problem is chronic muscle-tension headaches, you would be asked to simply relax while the measurement is taken of the muscles in the forehead. This measurement of the resting level is considered a starting point for training. You will gradually learn to control the forehead muscles so that the resting level after successful completion of eight to ten training sessions is greatly decreased when compared to initial pretraining resting levels.

Once a baseline has been established, it is time to begin biofeedback training. The basis of biofeedback is a process known as shaping. Shaping is a basic learning technique whereby progress towards an identified goal is accomplished through small, incremental steps. One step must be successfully mastered before proceeding to the next. Again using muscle-tension headaches as an example, reduced muscle activity or "tightness" is the ultimate goal of EMG biofeedback training. Therefore, your doctor or therapist sets a threshold for you so that a soft tone continuously sounds. Successful muscular relaxation will terminate the tone, thereby signalling that you have successfully decreased your muscle tension. A new threshold for you to work towards is set, and your job is to again terminate the tone by further relaxing your frontalis muscles. Step-by-step levels of muscle tension are decreased through shaping until the patient achieves a resting level of muscle tension which does not result in head pain.

After you begin to demonstrate moderate control of the targeted biological process, your doctor or therapist may introduce a voluntary control phase to the training protocol. During the voluntary control phase, you will *not* be given feedback. Rather, your doctor or therapist monitors your progress while you exert passive voluntary control of the targeted physiological process. Voluntary control phases instituted in the overall training protocol prohibit excessive dependence on continuous feedback to control biological processes and help generalize the patient's ability to control the targeted process outside of the doctor's office where continuous feedback is not available. When you are able to control successfully the targeted biological process during voluntary control phases, your doctor may ask you to begin practicing your control technique at home between training sessions.

After a number of biofeedback training sessions, which will vary depending on what type of [headache] you have and how quickly you learn, you should find that your ability to control the targeted response has increased while the time and effort required for voluntary control has decreased. The greater control you develop, the greater effect it should have on your [headaches]. While voluntary control of muscle activity may be relatively easy to learn, control of blood flow may take longer to accomplish and is somewhat more difficult for most people.

Exactly how does one go about learning voluntary control

of muscles or blood flow? If you asked most successful bio-feedback patients how they voluntarily exercise control over biological processes long thought to be involuntary, they would respond with, "I'm not sure!" Some report relaxing deeply while thinking of their body being warmed by a pene-trating heat. Others report conjuring up images of peaceful landscapes. The vast majority, however, report no specific sensation or thought. They describe successful biofeedback control as a "knack" or "sense" that is almost unconsciously produced. They describe it as "will" that, during early train-ing, requires deliberate and careful thought and effort but over time becomes a technique requiring very little con-sciousness.

Biofeedback with Chronic [Headaches]

Biofeedback is currently most widely recognized as effec-tive in the treatment of chronic-pain states. A review of the scientific literature evidences the use of biofeedback in the treatment of a variety of painful medical disorders with vary-ing degrees of success. At this time, it appears that biofeed-back training has proven most beneficial in the treatment of migraine and muscle-contraction headaches. . . . Let's take a closer look at how biofeedback is effectively utilized in the treatment of these troublesome chronic-pain disorders.

Migraine Headaches

Simply defined, migraine or vascular headache is a disorder characterized by excruciating pain usually located on one side of the head and often accompanied by nausea, vomiting, cognitive impairment, depression, and, occasionally, even suicidal thoughts. Migraine attacks are usually preceded by an aura of prodromal stage during which the victim experi-ences blurred or double vision, or even temporary blindness.

At times there are visions of bright flashing lights, strange shapes or dazzling colors.

A migraine attack usually comes in three states: prodromal, the actual attack and the aftermath. An attack may last anywhere from a few hours to several days, and the pain is nothing less than horrible. Twice as many women suffer migraine headaches as men and, although rare, migraines can affect children as well as adults. Many victims of migraine find that the attacks cease to occur when they reach middle age, although other victims endure migraines all their lives.

A fortunate discovery at the Menninger Foundation in Topeka, Kansas, in the late Sixties led to the development of the thermal biofeedback technique of treating migraine. During tests of the ability to learn control of blood flow to the extremities, a subject who happened to be experiencing a migraine at the time of the investigation reported an unexpected side effect. The subject claimed that she experienced a sudden decrease in the intensity and severity of her headache, which the researchers noted coincided with a dramatic increase in the blood flow to the subject's hands. This discovery was the catalyst for an intensive five-year study of thermal biofeedback as a treatment technique for migraine headaches.

Thermal biofeedback involves attaching a small, sensitive thermometer to the tip of the index finger. The thermometer measures the warmth of the skin, the skin temperature being associated with blood flow. In other words, the greater the warmth of the hands, as measured by a special thermometer, the greater the blood flow to the extremities. The patient is instructed to watch a meter that gives continuous visual feedback of hand temperature. Through trial-and-error practice and with instructions from the doctor or therapist, the patient soon learns to increase the warmth of the hands, thereby increasing the blood flow to the hands. After several training sessions, many patients learn to increase the warmth of their hands by as much as 8–10 °F (about 4 °C). Of course, voluntary control of extremity blood flow is associated with a decrease in frequency, intensity, and duration of migraine attacks.

Research and clinical results of thermal biofeedback effectiveness in the treatment of migraine headache have been mixed. While some studies report that as many as 60 to 80 percent of patients benefit from thermal biofeedback, perhaps a more accurate estimate may be closer to 40 or 50 percent. However, when thermal biofeedback is combined with relaxation exercises and modifications in life-style, the technique offers hope to many migraine victims who otherwise continue to suffer despite the best efforts of medical science.

Muscle-Contraction Headaches

The advertising world does not hesitate to suggest possible reasons and remedies for muscle-contraction (tension) headaches. We usually are shown a stress situation, such as a housewife rushing to prepare dinner while two or three children scream and cry, the telephone rings, the doorbell rings and the roast beef burns. The frantic housewife clutches her head in obvious distress as the television announcer recommends taking Brand X pills "for fast headache relief." In reality, this often does prove to be the case. Many of us are subject to occasional headaches when there is unusual pressure at home or work, when we are enduring a particularly frustrating period, or suffering from glare combined with heat. For this type of occasional head pain, "Brand X" analgesic pills probably work well. But what if the headaches occur more and more frequently, even daily, and the consumption of analgesics creeps up steadily? Medical attention is then usually required.

Tension headaches affect both sides of the head symmetrically in approximately 90 percent of tension-headache patients, unlike migraine which is usually located only on one side of the head. The quality of the headache is remarkably consistent and characteristic. It is often described as a tightness, more of an uncomfortable feeling of pressure than pain. It is also described as a dull ache in the forehead, or the temples, or the back of the head, or the neck, or even "all over the head." Approximately one in ten muscle-contraction-headache sufferers also is plagued with vascular involvement. Known as "combined muscle contraction–migraine" headaches, the disorder appears to be a link between the two maladies and frequently complicates an accurate diagnosis.

The victim of chronic tension headaches experiences pain not only during tense or stressful situations, but also may endure head pain in anticipation of any unpleasantness. The symptoms may later begin in advance of a day's work, a routine shopping trip, a visit to friends or any of the other aspects of daily life. In time, the patient's activity level and optimism decrease as the consumption of analgesic medication increases. The product is a distressing cycle of chronic pain and, as a result, further muscle tension and pain. Tense muscles cause pain because prolonged muscle constriction depletes the muscle of oxygen and decreases blood flow. As a result, toxins build up in muscle tissue, resulting in pain.

Biofeedback treatment of muscle-contraction headaches is based on the following premise: If muscular tension in the shoulders, neck and head can be decreased or prevented before it begins, and can be maintained at reduced levels, headache frequency can be reduced or even eliminated. Muscles give off electrical discharges which can be measured and recorded with biofeedback instruments. Electrodes are attached to the frontalis muscles in the forehead or to the neck and shoulders. The patient then uses continuous audio or visual feedback of muscle activity to learn techniques to reduce muscular tension. Specific relaxation exercises (Chapter 9) are frequently included as part of the treatment regimen, and successful elimination of tension headaches can usually be accomplished within five to ten training sessions. Once treatment ends, the patient must continue home practice of the relaxation technique to guard against relapse.

8

Massage

Massage and manipulation of the muscles in the face, head, neck and shoulders as practiced by masseurs, osteopaths, chiropractors, physical therapists or rank amateurs can produce a significant physical and psychological calming effect. More important to headache victims, many patients claim that massage can ease or even eliminate some attacks of headache. It seems that massage acts as a nonchemical tranquillizer, dispelling anxiety and relaxing tense muscles. In addition, massage stimulates both the surface skin and underlying tissues, improving circulation and triggering an increased supply of oxygen to the muscles and tissues. Most importantly, however, massage simply feels good. In the midst of a muscle-contraction headache, massage relaxes us and makes us feel better. During a migraine attack, massage acts much like relaxation exercises (Chapter 9), reducing our level of physiological and psychological reactivity and helping us to manage pain through muscular and cognitive relaxation.

Detractors of massage say it is little more than faith healing, the laying-on of hands practiced in the Middle Ages. They claim that no scientific theory or accepted research evidence exists to document the effectiveness of massage or warrant its use as a treatment modality. However, there is no doubt that massage does relax tense muscles, has a psychological calming effect, has no significant side effects and is recommended as a supplement to medical care.

In this chapter we will discuss how and why massage is an important component in the multimodal program for headache relief. Massage techniques for the face, scalp and trapezius muscles are easy to learn and take only a few minutes of practice each day. Massage should be done consistently at least once a day, and the key areas around the temples and ears, back of the head, and the neck and shoulders should be done several times daily, especially at the beginning of the program. We will conclude this chapter with a brief overview of the trigger points of acupressure, a technique still considered experimental, but one used by some practitioners in the control of pain.

FACE MASSAGE

There are several simple massage techniques that have often been found to be effective in relieving muscle-contraction headaches. Firm striking of the forehead is one. Grasp the headache victim's forehead as if it were a basketball, with the thumbs coming together at the hairline. Squeezing lightly with the other fingers, stroke towards the end of the forehead with the thumbs. In massage parlance, a stroke is more than just a light grazing movement. Firm, but not excessive pressure should be applied to the stroked area. Ideally, the skin of the forehead will be stretched just enough to make the patient's eyes close. Do not rub or apply friction. It takes a while to learn the difference between rubbing and deep stroking; you'll know you're pressing too hard or rubbing if you feel much resistance from the skin. Stroke all the way to the edge of the forehead, then slide your fingers gently over the skin to the original position and repeat this movement several times.

The same type of deep stroking applied to another area of the face can frequently help relieve both tension and sinus headaches. Join the thumbs at the tip of the nose with the fingers bunched together at the temples. Knead upward at the nose, the fingers moving up the temples to the hairline. When the thumbs reach the hollow between the eyes and the nose, stop kneading and make deep strokes with the thumbs moving over the eyebrows and towards the temples. Keep the fingers in place, exerting pressure at the top of the forehead. When you have completed this procedure, slide back to the original position and begin again.

After you have repeated the above technique several times, reposition the thumbs in the hollows under the eyes with the fingers at the temples. The bone structure that you feel about the cheeks and under the eyes is the infraorbital ridge. Stroke over the ridge to the tips of the eyebrows. Slide back and repeat the movement several times.

The next step is placing the thumbs over the bridge of the nose and the fingers at the temples. Knead upward in small circles to the hairline. Return the hands to a position close to the original one and repeat the movement, varying the position slightly until you have covered the entire forehead area.

When there is no one available to assist, you can perform the facial massage movements on yourself. Kneading the hollows between the eyes and nose can relieve pressure, as can general deep stroking of the forehead. Slight pressure on the temporal artery (above the cheekbone, next to the temple) for five or ten seconds every few minutes can sometimes give temporary relief from migraine headache.

SCALP MASSAGE

Scalp massage is also intended to stimulate blood flow and relax tense muscles; Figure 8-1 illustrates one such technique. Starting at the intersection of the forehead and temple, just above the eyebrow, press the fingertips against the skin and slowly work the fingers up the forehead towards the hairline. Just after working your way into the hair, begin to descend towards the earlobe. At that point, reverse back up in front of the ear, pass above the ear, and descend behind it, directly over the protusion of your skull behind the ear. This area at the lower back of the skull is important for headache sufferers since many large and small muscles pass from the neck to the skull. Unfortunately, many working positions (such as leaning over a desk, typewriter, workbench, sink, etc.) involve tipping the upper body forward so that the head is forward of the pelvis, or the head looks downward or both. When this is the case, the neck muscles must support the weight of the head in an unbalanced position, with resultant stress on the muscles. Since tensed and strained muscles can cause a headache, the base of the skull is a vitally important area. Massage it well and then return to the original position, starting again.

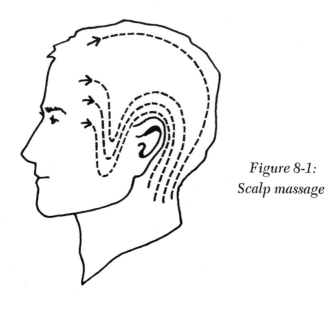

Figure 8-1:
Scalp massage

If you feel a headache coming on during the day and there is no one to assist you in massage exercises, you may perform much of the techniques yourself. For the side of the head, place your fingers together on the forehead and the thumbs will fall naturally in place. For the lower back of the head, place your knuckles directly over the ears and your thumbs will be in the proper place. Appendix B outlines some suggested face and scalp calisthenics which can be done throughout the day to help relax and tone these muscles.

TRAPEZIUS MASSAGE

The trapezius muscle (Figure 2-4) may be the most important muscle in the body as far as headaches are concerned. One important function of the trapezius is to hold the head erect. As mentioned previously, much of our work and leisure time is spent with the head tilted forward, placing a strain on the trapezius muscle. In addition, for many of us the trapezius seems a barometer of daily stress. During tense and stressful periods, it is not unusual to see someone with their shoulders hunched and drawn tight. The end result of faulty posture and/or stress is often a severe headache.

To massage the trapezius, place the fingertips on either side of the base of the skull and slowly knead the muscle while working down the neck and out each shoulder. Return to the original position, but this time press the thumbs into the muscle with a pressure just short of causing pain. Again, start at the base of the skull and work down the neck and out each shoulder. Finally, return to the original position and work out towards the shoulders, pinching the muscle between the fingers and thumb, being careful not to pinch too hard to cause pain. Simply "roll" the muscle between the fingertips and thumb. These exercises can be repeated as often as you wish. Appendix C outlines some neck and shoulder calisthenics that can be performed throughout the day to keep the trapezius muscle relaxed and comfortable.

ACUPRESSURE

Although acupuncture (puncturing the skin with needles) and acupressure (applying pressure with a finger to selected areas of the body) have been in use in the Far East for thousands of years, they have only recently become more popular in other parts of the world. Various points along the body have been identified and termed "meridians," which are thought to interact with other body parts. Western investigations have identified these same acupressure points by measuring the electrical resistance of the skin. For example, normal dry skin will show a surface resistance of about 500,000 ohms, although the resistance will vary with perspiration and

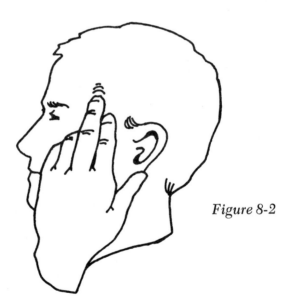

Figure 8-2

Feel for the depression in the skull located behind the eyebrow on both sides of the head.

other factors. But as the skin is tested point by point, certain small areas are identified where the electrical resistance is only 12,000 to 15,000 ohms. These points turn out to be the

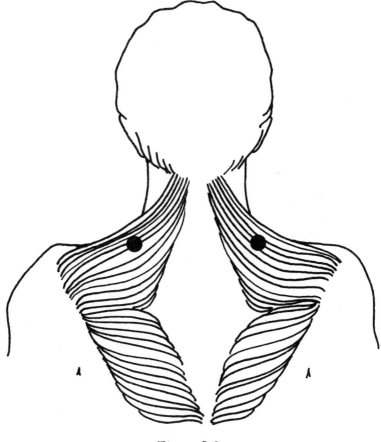

Figure 8-3

traditional acupuncture or acupressure points. Proponents of acupuncture and acupressure believe that stimulation of these points produces therapeutic changes in body functioning and health.

Western theoretical explanations for these points remain poorly developed, and although some practitioners and pain clinics utilize acupressure extensively, the technique generally remains experimental and of questionable effectiveness. However, a number of patients, including headache victims, report receiving some benefit from acupressure. For those interested in the location of headache meridian points, several have been included below.

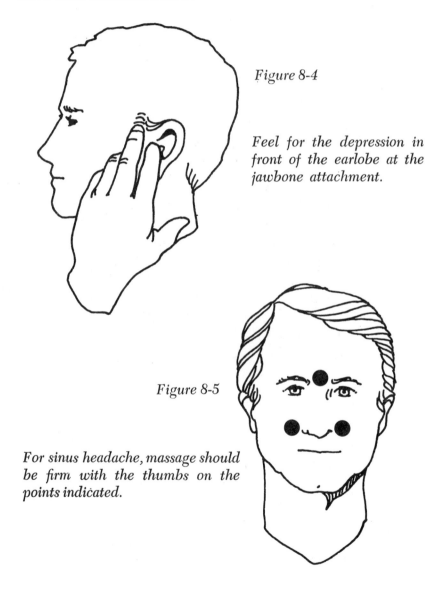

Figure 8-4

Feel for the depression in front of the earlobe at the jawbone attachment.

Figure 8-5

For sinus headache, massage should be firm with the thumbs on the points indicated.

9

Hypnosis and Relaxation

Relaxation of the body and mind is an integral part of the multimodal approach to headache relief. It has long been known that anxiety expressed as muscular tension and a "busy mind" functions as part of what can be termed the "feedback loop of pain" (Figure 9-1). In other words, pain that results from headache is a negative sensation that carries an increase in physiological (muscle) and cognitive (mental) arousal. For the purposes of this discussion, heightened physiological and cognitive arousal can be termed anxiety. Anxiety, in turn, causes an uncomfortable increase in muscular tension and mental distress which serves to increase the intensity of pain.

The feedback loop of pain is a natural involuntary response to the noxious perception of pain. To break this snowball effect, you must learn to relax. Sounds simple? Unfortunately, relaxation in general—and particularly in the face of pain— is not so simple. Deep and effective relaxation is a skill that, like other skills, must be perfected through proper technique and practice. In this chapter we shall first study how to utilize effective relaxation to decrease the frequency and intensity of headaches and then examine the role of hypnosis, a special type of relaxation, in headache relief.

RELAXATION

For our purposes we can consider relaxation the opposite of tension. Most people readily assume that one flourishes in the absence of the other; that is, if you're not tense, you must be relaxed. Unfortunately, the human body does not function that simply. If you consider relaxation positioned on one end of a continuum and tension on the other, there is a huge grey area in between where we all exist most of the time. A typical day may have some moments of tension and some of relaxation, most of us existing in a kind of psychic limbo. Yet it is often that tension is building within us. Stimuli too small to be consciously registered are tightening our muscles, aggravating our nerves and constricting our blood vessels. At the end of the day there will be a blinding headache, with no apparent cause.

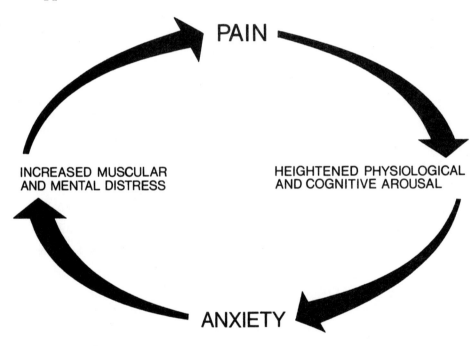

Figure 9-1: Feedback loop of pain

Relaxation cannot be building quietly in our bodies as we go through a routine day because so much stress exists in our lives. To combat the negative effects, one must learn to relax. Simply defined, relaxation is the absence of mental and physical stress which is achieved when the body is in equilibrium and the mind is unhampered by anxiety. It is physiologically impossible and psychologically impractical for an individual to be always relaxed, since the mind thrives on a certain amount of controlled, creative turbulence. It is, however, feasible for each of us to be able to control bodily processes enough to regulate the energy and excitation flow of the system.

The ability to relax can have a dramatic effect on headaches. Amazing physiological changes occur in the relaxed body; heartbeat and respiration slow, and the quality of electrical waves in the brain changes. Alpha waves, which can be recorded from the brain during peaceful, tranquil moments when the eyes are closed, become more numerous. Research conducted at the Johns Hopkins Headache Clinic in Baltimore, Maryland, suggest that using biofeedback to teach subjects to increase the percentage of alpha waves from the brain could often reduce headache frequency. Muscles also loosen and lengthen during relaxation.

Physiological relaxation most often leads to cognitive or psychological relaxation. The emotions are tranquil, and a feeling of peace prevails. Western scientists have found that the simple process of meditation, thought by many to be a form of relaxation, can have wide-reaching physiological effects. Studies conducted on Zen monks in Japan showed that during meditation, the monks were able to decrease their consumption of oxygen and output of carbon dioxide by approximately twenty percent. Slowdowns in heartbeat and respiration have also been observed in yoga practitioners. All of this leads to a deceleration in metabolism, a tranquillizing of the emotional state, a reduction in tension and a decrease in the incidence of headaches.

Learning to Relax

Relaxation is a skill that can be learned and perfected with practice. One particularly effective and popular relaxation technique is known as *progressive muscular relaxation* and involves practicing exercises that mechanically manipulate the skeletal muscles of the entire body into a more relaxed state. In the early 1900s, Dr. Edmond Jacobson* first outlined the principles of progressive muscular relaxation, and the exercises have since been modified numerous times. Once the basic relaxation technique is learned, it is vital that the technique be practiced. With serious practice, less time is required to achieve the desired stage of deep relaxation. The technique can then be used to ward off headaches, reduce stress, assist in sleep and to decrease the intensity of headache pain. The following procedure and technique are recommended.

Procedure:

1. When first learning to relax, a quiet, dimly lit place is an ideal one in which to practice.
2. Lie on your back on a carpeted floor or sit in a comfortable chair. Avoid practicing relaxation exercises in bed since most mattresses do not provide sufficient support.
3. Try to eliminate all other competing thoughts from your mind. Relaxation exercises are intended to relax your body *and* your mind.
4. Focus all attention on the muscle group being tensed.
5. Tense muscle groups on cue. Get in a habit of following the same procedure each time you practice relaxation exercises.
6. Hold the tension and focus all attention on the buildup of tension in every muscle group for six to ten seconds.

*Dr. Jacobson was the founder of the Laboratory of Clinical Physiology in Chicago, Illinois.

7. Release the tension from each muscle group all at once. Do *not* gradually relax a muscle group at the end of six to ten seconds, but instead let the muscle relax suddenly, as if turning off a light switch.
8. After relaxing a muscle group, focus all of your attention on relaxation for twenty to thirty seconds. Concentrate on the different sensation between tension and relaxation.
9. Repeat for each muscle group.
10. Practice relaxation exercises at least twice daily, but the more the better!

Technique:

1. Lie on your back on the floor. Make a tight fist and tense the muscles of the forearm of the right hand and arm. Imagine you are holding a golf ball in the palm of the right hand and squeezing it. Relax.
2. Make a tight fist, bending the right arm at the elbow and tensing the muscles of the upper arm. Relax.
3. Make a tight fist and tense the muscles of the forearm of the left hand and arm. Imagine you are holding a golf ball in the palm of the left hand and squeezing it. Relax.
4. Make a tight fist, bending the left arm at the elbow and tensing the muscles of the upper arm. Relax.
5. Tense the muscles of the neck. Push your chin towards your chest, and pulling your head at the same time, lift your head off the floor. Relax.
6. Tense the muscles of your face. Clamp your jaw tightly shut and pull back on the corners of the mouth. Squint your eyes tightly shut and wrinkle your nose. Raise your eyebrows towards your hairline and wrinkle your forehead. Relax.
7. Tense the muscles of your shoulders, chest and back. Take a deep breath and hold it. Now pull the shoulders back and together much like the military attention posture. Relax.

8. Tense the muscle of the abdomen. Take a deep breath and bear down with the stomach muscles. Relax.
9. Tense the muscles of the buttocks and right thigh. Press the back of the right knee down into the floor. Relax.
10. Tense the muscles of the right calf and foot. Bend the foot at the ankle and stretch the toes towards the head. Relax.
11. Tense the muscles of the buttocks and left thigh. Press the back of the left knee down into the floor. Relax.
12. Tense the muscles of the left calf and foot. Bend the foot at the ankle and stretch the toes towards the head. Relax.

When you have completed this exercise, take two to three deep breaths and hold each one for a moment, deeply relaxing as you exhale. Enjoy this relaxed state, breathing regularly and slowly to enhance it. Imagery has been found to occur when an individual feels deeply relaxed; if you experience pleasant imagery, allow it to continue and focus on it. When you are ready to end the exercise, slowly count backwards from five to one. Move slowly until fully alert. The key to managing your headaches by achieving deep muscular relaxation is to practice continually.

NOTE: The above-described relaxation exercise is only one of many relaxation techniques designed to reduce muscle tension. While relaxation techniques are very useful, they should not serve as substitutes for professional health care. See your doctor if you have difficulty learning this technique, if it does not seem to be reducing your tension levels or if your body feels relaxed but your mind continues to race.

HYPNOSIS

Hypnosis has in recent years gradually gained more acceptance as a useful medical and psychological treatment technique.* Perhaps the most effective use of hypnosis in the treatment of headaches and other pain states is physiological and psychological relaxation. Hypnosis has been found to facilitate decreased physiological arousal and is an excellent relaxation technique. Research has shown hypnosis to be effective in the treatment of pain associated with such disorders as burns, anxiety, cancer, tension, arthritis, leukemia, menstrual discomfort, ulcers, postoperative pain and nausea, childbirth, neck and lower back pain, dental procedures and headaches.

The Hypnotic Experience

The hypnotic experience can best be thought of as a continuum, ranging from a very light state which we can drift into without even being aware of it, to the deepest stages which may appear similar to a sleepwalker's state of consciousness. The lightest stages of hypnosis seem almost like a game that the brain plays on us. Perhaps you can remember times when your gaze seemed drawn to some blank wall or even into space and your mind seemed totally blank. Maybe your breathing became full and slow, your heart rate decreased and your muscles seemed unusually relaxed. You felt calm, tranquil and totally at peace.

When you snapped back to reality you felt as if you had been a million miles from earth, although you remembered exactly what you were thinking and feeling. The feeling is similar to that sensation experienced just before falling asleep, except that rather than feeling dulled and hazy, our concentration seems crystal clear!

The middle or intermediate stage of hypnosis is characterized by the increased intensity of those sensations experienced in the lightest stage. The body feels even more

*Pages 98–102 are excerpted from *Managing Chronic Pain: A Patient's Guide*, pp. 82–84.

peaceful and relaxed, while the mind seems more alert and clearer than ever. During this stage we also become more susceptible to suggestion. The body and mind seem free from the limitations of everyday living, and we are more fully able to achieve our true physical and mental capabilities. Frequently, we find that an arm or leg can be extended for prolonged periods of time without strain or fatigue. We may even sense that time has stopped, or is speeding rapidly by; that a stationary object is moving, or that a once painful area of the body is now less painful or pain-free.

Individuals susceptible to the intermediate stage of hypnosis will often report being completely aware of what they were doing and feeling unusually calm, relaxed and confident that they could achieve whatever the hypnotist suggested. These individuals frequently report a feeling of confidence that they could bring themselves out of the hypnotic state at will.

The deepest stage of hypnosis is sometimes termed somnambulism and is best described as similar to a sleepwalker's state of consciousness. This stage is characterized by an even more powerful intensity of those perceptual and physical sensations common in the light and intermediate stages of hypnosis. For example, in the deepest stage of hypnosis, mental acuity may be so concentrated as to enable the person to recall past events that have long been forgotten or suppressed. The technique of age regression, so popular in the media, can occasionally be accomplished in the somnambulistic stage. Needless to say, susceptibility to suggestion is greatly enhanced in the deepest stage, and individuals returning to normal consciousness from somnambulistic hypnosis occasionally report no memory of their thoughts or actions during the session. It is generally agreed that only about one in ten individuals is susceptible to the somnambulistic stage.

It is important to understand that the stages of hypnosis are not as clearly defined as this presentation may appear. While in a light stage of hypnosis, some individuals experience the perceptual and physical sensations common in the deepest stage. Again, it is best that one think of hypnosis as a flexible continuum rather than as three separate and distinct stages and realize that the therapeutic effects of hypnosis do not depend on the depth of the hypnotic state. Many individuals are able to relax deeply while in a light hypnotic stage.

How Hypnosis Works

As mentioned, no one knows exactly how hypnosis works, but we do know three general components that appear to be most important in successful hypnosis: concentration, suggestibility and imagination. Successful hypnotic induction depends, to a great extent, on the voluntary cooperation of the patient who is asked to concentrate intently on the suggestions of the doctor. The ability to concentrate deeply varies among individuals, but it is most likely to be found in people who readily accept the fact that there are several states of consciousness. How well can you concentrate? Are you able to shut out the distractions of the day when you go to bed at night? Can you read a book in a noisy dorm or when the television is blaring?

A second important component of hypnosis may be termed suggestibility—meaning that hypnosis tends to be most effective if you expect it to be. Some people feel that suggestibility is a negative trait. Perhaps they equate being suggestible with being naive or gullible. This is unfortunate, for suggestibility is a positive and important trait in hypnosis.

During hypnosis the patient may receive a suggestion from the doctor that he is engaged in some other mental or physical activity that is incompatible with the problem behavior.

To illustrate, let's imagine a patient with [headaches described as tightness around the head with pain up the back of the neck]. During hypnosis, the doctor may suggest that the patient is experiencing a warm, relaxed feeling through the neck and head rather than [tight, constricting pain]. As the neck and head warm, the pain gradually subsides, and the experience of pain is replaced by an experience of relaxed warmth. Though the patient's central nervous system continues to receive pain impulses, his concentration has been diverted to the feelings of warmth and muscle relaxation. Remember, pain exists only if it is perceived!

A third component of hypnosis is imagination. Do you have a vivid and strong imagination? If you were asked to sit quietly, close your eyes, and imagine floating high above the ground on a giant, pillowy white cloud, could you do it? Would you feel the texture of the cloud against your skin? Would you look far below and see the green treetops and the colors of the landscape? Would you close your eyes and feel a warm breeze gently blowing your cloud across the sky? The ability to create rich, vivid mental images may be more closely related to hypnotic susceptibility than any other characteristic.

In summary, research suggests that those who benefit most from hypnosis tend to be able to concentrate well and are suggestible, imaginative and truly motivated to seek relief from their pain. Is this an accurate description of you? If so, then the chances are excellent that you will be a good candidate for hypnotic pain control.

10
Diet

Dietary habits have been suspected of playing an important contributing role in attacks of head pain since the early writings of the Roman physician Galen. Some 2,000 years later, the exact association between headaches and diet remains unclear, but modern research appears to point a suspecting finger at certain foods which are thought to act as a triggering mechanism for vascular headaches. Dr. John Fothergill was an early advocate of the suspected link between certain foods and headaches. Writing in 1778, Dr. Fothergill claimed, "It is most clear that the headache proceeds from the stomach, not the reverse."* He blamed certain foods, particularly "melted butter, fat meats, spices, meat pies, hot buttered toast, and malted liquors when strong and hoppy." Dr. Fothergill went on to add, "From many incontestible proofs that butter in considerable quantity is injurius, it is less used in many families. Nothing more speedily and effectively gives the sick-headache, and sometimes within a few hours."

The food-sensitivity theory of migraine headaches is a controversial one. Many authorities are convinced that certain foods induce migraine attacks in susceptible individuals (see Appendix A). The foods most frequently mentioned are

*G. Shelby and J. W. Lance, "Observations on 500 Cases of Migraine," *Journal of Neurology, Neurosurgery and Psychiatry*, Vol. 23 (1960), p. 66.

chocolate, fried or fatty foods, frankfurters, salami, bologna, cocoa, onions, peanuts, cheese, oranges and Chinese food. Other authorities point to a lack of conclusive research evidence identifying certain foods with the onset of headaches. For example, Dr. Harold G. Wolff, a noted pioneer in headache research, reported some years ago that "with the administration of chocolate disguised in capsules for those allegedly sensitive to chocolate, or milk given through a stomach tube to those who are said to be sensitive to milk, the results did not confirm an association between these foods and headache attacks."* Dr. Edda Hanington, a British physician, and A. Murray Harper, a physiologist, later countered by reporting that tyramine, which is present in cheese and eggs, could produce a migraine in susceptible individuals.* However, a more recent replication of this experiment did not confirm the association between cheese and eggs (tyramine) and migraine headaches.

Beer and wine have also been suspected of being catalysts for the development of migraine headaches. Interestingly, both beer and wine also contain tyramine. Dr. Hanington comments, "When a susceptible patient eats foods containing tyramine or drinks beer or wine, the following chain of events is set in motion: Tyramine releases norepinephrine (an adrenal hormone) from tissues within the brain, which causes the blood vessels of the brain and scalp to constrict. At this point the visual disturbances marking the onset of migraine appear. When the supply of norepinephrine is exhausted, the scalp vessels rebound from the constriction by dilating, which causes the intense head pain. The headache finally ceases when the tissue stores of norepinephrine have been replenished."†

Sufficient experimentation has now been conducted to con-

*H. G. Wolff, *Headache and Other Head Pain*, 3rd ed. (London: Oxford University Press, 1972), p. 310.

†Ibid., p. 409.

firm Dr. Hanington's belief that tyramine can act as a migraine-precipitating agent in certain susceptible headache sufferers. It is also suspected that women sensitive to tyramine can experience migraines if they take oral contraceptives. This is because the enzyme that breaks down tyramine in the body is inhibited by the chemical action of the contraceptives, thereby allowing vascular constriction to take place. Many women with no previous history of headaches report the onset of migraines after they begin taking birth control pills.

Dr. Hanington's search into the role of tyramine and food sensitivity in precipitating migraine attacks has added much to our understanding of diet and health. Part of this research involves the compilation of a list of foods that Dr. Hanington believes must be avoided by the migraine-susceptible individual. Each of the following foods listed in order of frequency was implicated in the migraine attacks experienced by 250 patients involved in a research investigation.*

Food	Percent
chocolate	72
dairy products	47
citrus fruits	32
alcohol	25
fatty fried foods	18
vegetables (onions)	18
tea and coffee	15
pork	14
seafood	10

It should be noted that research evidence identifying the above foods with the onset of migraine attacks is neither conclusive nor universally accepted. Even Dr. Hanington acknowledges that dietary factors are reported by only one-third

*How Foods Give Entree to Migraine, p. 77.

of all migraine patients. Nevertheless, if you are a victim of migraine, the minimal efforts required to avoid the above-mentioned foods are worthwhile, given a chance at headache relief. First, chart the number of headaches you have during the next thirty days while on your regular diet. Next, alter your diet for thirty days to completely avoid the foods mentioned as precipitating migraines. Compare the recording charts to see if diet control made a difference in your headache frequency.

NUTRITION AND HEALTH

While the cause-and-effect relationship of certain foods and headaches remains a topic of scientific debate, there is little question that an inadequate diet makes the body susceptible to all kinds of illnesses, including headaches. We often eat too much (especially fats and sugar), and distribute the intake poorly throughout the day. A prudent daily diet involves three or four small meals that consist of a balanced combination of *resistance* foods and minimal amounts of *susceptibility* foods. Resistance foods are those whose consumption has been found to increase resistance to illness and disease. Included in this food group are whole grain products, vegetables, fruits and animal products. Susceptibility foods are those whose consumption has been observed to increase susceptibility to illness and disease, including headaches; these foods include salt, alcoholic beverages, refined grain products, sugar products and caffeine-containing foods.

Resistance Foods

Vegetables. Vegetables are an important source of vitamins, minerals and fibre. One raw salad should be eaten daily. A large salad is an excellent way to start the evening meal. Read the labels on frozen or canned vegetables: They should not contain fat, sauces, cheese, glazes or similar seasonings. Since ingredients are labelled in descending order of predominance, avoid those in which corn sweetener or syrup, sugar or salt are listed among the first few ingredients. Preparation of vegetable casseroles will aid in using a variety of vegetables and may replace a meat entree.

Fruits. Fruits satisfy your sweet tooth but do not add refined sugar to your diet; consequently, they are known as "natural" desserts. They can be used in salads, for snacks and in the lunch box. Like vegetables, they are valuable sources of vitamins, minerals and fibre. Raw fruits are best; however, those canned in their own juice, unsweetened or artificially sweetened, are acceptable. When buying frozen fruits, select the "loose pack," not those frozen in syrup. Fruits are preferred to fruit juices because blood sugar levels remain more stable, and fruits contain more nutrients and fibre.

Bread and cereal products. Whole grain breads and crackers are recommended; these may be homemade or commercial. Labels of commercial breads should be checked carefully to see whether whole grain flour is the principal ingredient. While it is rarely possible to find commercial breads not containing sucrose (sugar), honey or molasses, these should not be the principal ingredients. When available, select breads containing oils rather than butter. Wheat germ, brewer's yeast, wheat and rice bran and polishings are valuable sources of nutrients, especially the trace minerals. The bran and polishings are also superior sources of plant fibre, which is potentially of great value for the well-being of the intestinal tract. These can be added to breads, cereals and other foods.

Plant fibre. Fibre is probably the single most neglected resistance food component in the American diet. It is the carbohydrate portion of grains, vegetables and fruits which is not digested by the human intestinal tract. Restoring fibre intake is reported to improve bowel function, possibly reduce the likelihood of colon cancer, and possibly prevent the development of hemorrhoids and diverticula.

Protein foods. The basic building blocks for all protein are the amino acids. The basic dietary building blocks used by the body to manufacture protein are nine essential amino acids (those amino acids the body cannot make itself in the process of building protein molecules from amino acids). For this building process to occur, all nine amino acids must be consumed together; otherwise, they are simply used as energy-like carbohydrates and fat. The ideal amino acid pattern for man is found in milk, followed closely by eggs. The next most nearly perfect pattern is other animal proteins, followed closely by soy protein and other plant proteins.

By learning to combine proteins from different plant families (for example, beans and grains), the complete essential amino acid pattern can be achieved. Animal protein is the highest quality protein, but it is usually found in association with significant amounts of saturated fats—and no fibre. Plant protein, on the other hand, is not as complete in terms of essential amino acids. However, sources of plant protein are high in fibre and their fat is primarily of the unsaturated type.

Eating very small servings of meat, combined with plant proteins, is a good way to get the essential amino acids. The meat flavor enhances the taste of vegetables, while the consumption of fat is minimized.

Susceptibility Foods

Modifying your dietary habits is not as hard as you may think. A balanced diet provides for generous amounts of appetite-satisfying starch and fibre. Many headache patients are convinced they feel much better when they adhere to a nutritious diet.

Sugar. Sugar, the most widely used food additive in the United States, adds "empty" calories to foods of all sorts, ranging from hot dogs to canned peas. The average American consumes about 135 pounds of sugar per year; this amount represents 670 calories daily, or one-third the recommended daily calories for an adult woman.

Alcoholic beverages. Like sugar, alcoholic beverages deplete the body stores of vitamins and minerals and are empty calories. In addition, as previously noted, alcohol is suspected by many individuals to be a precipitating factor in attacks of migraine headaches.

Caffeine-containing foods. These should be used sparingly. Examples of such foods are coffee, tea and cola drinks. In addition to its effect as a central-nervous-system stimulant, caffeine increases blood sugar levels. Abstinence or limited consumption of caffeine-containing foods has been suggested for individuals with high or low blood sugar problems. It is also suggested that coffee drinkers use decaffeinated coffee.

Salt. Almost everyone would benefit from a reduction in salt intake; it is mandatory for those with high blood pressure and for those who retain fluid in their bodies. The average American uses almost two teaspoons of salt a day. Next to sugar, salt is the most widely used food additive. The actual need for salt is less than one-fourth of a gram. (Seven grams equal one teaspoon.) A maximum of five grams per day has been recommended. This modest reduction requires only that a person avoid salty foods and the use of added salt.

A properly balanced diet is essential to your general health whether or not such a diet has any effect on your headaches. Should your selection of foods result in a decrease in headaches, you are a two-time winner!

HYPOGLYCEMIA AND HEADACHES

If you wake up with head pain in the middle of the night, have morning headaches or consistently experience headaches in the late afternoon, you should consider the possibility that you may be hypoglycemic. Though probably less common than recently emphasized, hypoglycemia is a medical disorder in which the body's normal balance of blood sugar levels is impaired and, as a result, blood sugar levels drop. In an over-simplified sense, hypoglycemia is the opposite of diabetes. In diabetes, blood sugar rises above normal levels; in hypoglycemia, the blood sugar level drops to a point where the body cannot function properly.

Since blood sugar levels are partly dependent on the intake of proper foods, many hypoglycemic patients will experience headaches several hours after a meal. This is the time when the stomach empties and the body's supply of glucose (simple sugar) runs low. Other than headaches, symptoms of hypoglycemia often include dizziness, irritability, nervousness, unusual fatigue, sleep problems in which you wake and can't go back to sleep, tremors, cold sweats, anxiety and/or depression and muscle pains.

If you frequently experience some of these symptoms, consult your physician. If he feels that hypoglycemia is a possibility, he will likely schedule you for a glucose tolerance test. This test involves taking multiple blood samples to determine blood sugar levels after you ingest a special sugar compound. If it turns out that you are hypoglycemic, your doctor will probably suggest a special diet in order to better balance the blood sugar levels in your body.

Suggested Foods

A diet for hypoglycemics generally consists of foods high in complete protein and fats, low in sugars and very low amounts of starches. Poultry, fish, lean meats and eggs are good. Fresh fruits (except citrus fruits which should be eaten in moderation) provide a number of important vitamins. Vegetables such as tomatoes, squash and cucumbers are beneficial, as are soybeans, nuts and peanut butter. For snacks, yogurt is frequently recommended for hypoglycemic patients.

Foods to Avoid

Cookies, cakes, pies, pastries, potato chips, ice cream, cola drinks, sugar-sweetened soft drinks and other sweet snack foods are most definitely to be avoided as are sugar-sweetened juices, canned or frozen fruits and vegetables packed in sugar-sweetened liquids. In the vegetable family, corn, lima beans, baked beans and potatoes are not recommended; neither is rice. Coffee, tea and, most importantly, all alcoholic beverages should be deleted from the hypoglycemic's diet altogether.

For further information about hypoglycemia, consult your physician or write to the Hypoglycemia Foundation, P.O. Box 98, Fleetwood, Mt. Vernon, New York 10552.

11

Physical Conditioning

Physical exercise occupies a special and important place in the multimodal program for headache relief. Muscle-contraction headaches are caused by tight and tense muscles, and some researchers believe that stress and tension play some precipitating role in migraine attacks. Headache pain and the fear of another attack of headache often cause the headache sufferer to become withdrawn and frequently avoid any activity which is thought may trigger another attack of pain. A proper program of graduated physical conditioning, however, can provide numerous therapeutic benefits.

EXERCISE AND HEALTH

The concept of physical conditioning has recently been popularized among laymen and professionals because of research documenting the beneficial effects of a proper exercise program. An increasing number of researchers emphasize the importance of conditioning in both physical and mental health. In this section we will briefly review some of the advantages of a proper conditioning program. As you will see, exercise has a therapeutic effect on the entire body, as well as relieving stress and relaxing tense "headache" muscles.

The Mind

Exercise, it seems, is often an effective and healthy nonchemical tranquillizer. In a study conducted at Purdue University in Lafayette, Indiana, sixty middle-aged faculty and staff members, all of them employed in sedentary jobs, participated in a four-month exercise program. Their personalities were evaluated both before and after the program, using a standard test known as the Cattell 16 Personality Factor Questionnaire. As they became better physically conditioned, the subjects were found to become more emotionally stable, more self-sufficient, more imaginative and more confident.

Dr. Richard Driscoll of Eastern State Psychiatric Hospital in Knoxville, Tennessee, also found that regular exercise makes people less anxious, particularly if they think pleasant thoughts during the workout. Dr. Michael B. Mock of the National Heart, Lung and Blood Institute reports that exercise has been found to counteract depressed feelings by increasing one's feeling of self-esteem and independence.

Dr. John Griest of the University of Wisconsin recently reported some rather startling investigative results. Dr. Greist assigned patients suffering from depression to either a ten-week exercise program or ten weeks of traditional psychotherapy. The results of his study suggest that the exercise program was more effective in alleviating depression. While there are numerous methodological flaws in some of the research cited, the general suggestion is clear: A regular program of exercise has a positive effect on our personalities.

Dr. Hans Selye of the University of Montreal has been studying stress for four decades. He believes that each of us possesses at birth a given amount of what he calls adaptation energy. When that energy is depleted, we experience a mental or physical breakdown. One way to avoid such a breakdown is by deliberately directing stress at varying body systems. Dr. Selye believes that a voluntary change of activity is as good or even better than rest. For example, when fatigued at the end of a long, tough day at the office, it is better to rigorously exercise for 30 minutes than to take a short nap.

Substituting demands on our musculature for those previously made on the intellect not only gives our brain a rest, but it helps to relax the body as well. Dr. Selye believes that stress on one body system helps to relax another.

The Nerves

Nerves benefit from physical conditioning by becoming more efficient at transmitting electrochemical impulses and activating more muscle fibres, thereby increasing strength. Furthermore, as reflexes replace voluntary actions, movement becomes more efficient. Wasteful muscular contractions become fewer, unneeded muscles relax more fully and movement is simplified. In short, the body becomes a more efficient and productive machine.

The Muscles

With proper physical conditioning, muscles stretch and become stronger. With consistent exercise, changes occur within the cells of our muscles. As cells change, so do muscle fibres. Muscle contraction is both faster and stronger. Furthermore, because the muscle fibres don't tire as easily, work can continue longer, and you may find yourself less fatigued at the end of a long day; you may feel stronger, more limber and refreshed.

The Blood

Embraced by hemoglobin, blood travels throughout our bodies delivering oxygen to the muscles. To increase the blood's efficiency as exercise begins, fluid leaves the bloodstream and fills small cavities betwen muscle cells. This serves two important purposes. First, the muscles work more smoothly and easily when bathed in fluid; second, the blood's hemoglobin concentration rises, allowing a given volume of blood to transport more oxygen than usual.

With a regular program of physical conditioning, an important change takes place in the blood: The body, in effect learning to expect its blood volume to be periodically lowered, increases its supply. Consequently, when fluid leaves the bloodstream at the onset of exercise, a larger quantity remains to carry out essential tasks.

With a consistent program of exercise, the composition of the blood is changed in still other ways. For example, its clotting ability is enhanced. Furthermore, since clots, once formed, must be dissolved, an enzyme called fibrinolysin appears in greater quantities. At the same time, certain lipids —such as the types of cholesterol and triglycerides associated with heart disease—become less concentrated in the blood.

The Heart

Few effects of physical conditioning have been more thoroughly documented than those that occur within the heart. Research has demonstrated that with proper conditioning the heart becomes a distinctly more efficient instrument, capable of doing more while working less hard. One of the most fundamental changes that occurs is the lengthening of the heart muscle fibres; a similar process occurs in the lengthening of leg muscles when we do stretching exercises. Longer fibres allow the heart's chambers to pump more blood with each contraction. As a result, the heart rate slows since the heart becomes more efficient. In addition, blood pressure during rest is usually reduced. Since high blood pressure is known to contribute to heart attacks, a lowering of the blood pressure is a welcomed benefit of exercise.

We have briefly reviewed just a few of the many advantages of a proper program of physical conditioning. While no unequivocal scientific data exists to date, most physicians believe that proper physical conditioning prolongs life. Even if the life span is not expanded, there is little argument that the quality of life is enhanced by exercise. Physical conditioning relieves stress, relaxes tense muscles, improves endurance and vascular blood flow—all of which are associated in some way with the most common varieties of headaches.

A PROGRAM FOR PHYSICAL CONDITIONING

The first step in planning a program to become better physically conditioned is simple: Consult your physician. Your physician should approve not only your participation in an exercise program, but the type of conditioning program as well.

The second step is to set realistic goals. A 40-year-old office manager in poor physical condition who has spent years behind a desk cannot realistically expect to be a marathon runner overnight. In fact, depending on your age, health and physical condition, perhaps even light jogging is unrealistic, particularly during the early stages of training. Brisk walking is in this case a more realistic and healthy form of exercise.

It is also important to keep your expectations for progress realistic. Rather than being goal-oriented and setting expectations for distance, time and endurance, exercise at a leisurely pace and let progress occur naturally. Setting expectations is not conducive to relaxation and can make exercise stressful and laborious. Your goal is not to enter the Olympics, but to improve your health. Allow your exercise programs to be relaxing and enjoyable.

The third step in improved physical conditioning is to include five minutes of stretching and limbering exercises before beginning more rigorous exercises, since tension and stress contract muscles and sudden physical exertion can result in "pulled" muscles and pain. It is also a good idea to practice a few minutes of stretching exercises at various times throughout the day. Keeping your muscles loose and relaxed may help avoid the onset of tension headaches throughout the day.

The final step is to plan your daily exercise program at a specific time and to work out regularly. Many well-intentioned people have attempted to "squeeze in" an exercise program between their busy daily routines, only to find themselves completing routines but failing to exercise or perhaps exercising only once a week. If you are serious about getting the benefits of physical conditioning, you must exercise *at least* every other day, preferably daily. Physical conditioning should become as much a part of your life as eating, sleeping and working. The multimodal program for headache relief is not easy, as it requires that you work with your physician and assume an active role and responsibility for your health. If you are willing to accept the challenge, physical conditioning is one component of the five-part multimodal program which can make a difference in your health.

12

A Daily Plan for Headache Relief

The multimodal program for headache relief is based in large part on altering maladaptive life-styles, which for our purposes we can define as life-styles abounding with tension, stress, deadlines and goals but short on relaxation, recreation and physical conditioning. Many of us are guilty of living what we have just defined as maladaptive life-styles, and our health suffers as a result: We suffer with headaches, heart disease, emotional problems, ulcers or a host of other health problems thought by many to be stress-related. So why don't we heed the warnings of contemporary scientists who repeatedly point an accusing finger at the negative effects of stress? While there may be many complex answers, in recent years the field of behavioral psychology has accumulated a significant amount of research which serves to clarify the roles of reinforcement and aversion in shaping our behavior.

Behavioral psychology tells us that much of our behavior, be it "adaptive" or "maladaptive," is shaped by reinforcement. For example, children may be disruptive at home because their behavior elicits the attention of an otherwise nonattentive parent. To such a child, it does not matter that the attention (a spanking, for example) may be negative. Sometimes even the negative consequences of acting out are better than no attention at all, so the child continues engaging in disruptive behavior.

According to another psychological theory, if a maladaptive behavior or life-style is to be modified, negative consequences or punishment must be delivered contingent on the behavior and must be delivered immediately following the behavior. Perhaps this is why some people continue to smoke cigarettes despite the fact that the Surgeon General of the United States has determined that cigarette smoking is dangerous to one's health. Cancer and heart disease, which may develop as consequences of smoking, are not diagnosed immediately, generally taking years of cardiopulmonary abuse. If we suffered a heart attack immediately after lighting a cigarette, the incidence of smoking would decrease drastically. The same can be said of eating too much, another health hazard. Rather than slowly creeping up the scale if we gained ten pounds immediately after overindulging, many sweet and rich foods would quickly disappear from most menus.

If we apply the above psychological theory to stressful life-styles and behaviors which often result in headache, we begin to better see our responsibility in an effort to modify headaches. First, many headache victims live by the clock: Deadlines must be met, work must be completed and goals must be achieved in record time. These individuals are described by many doctors as being "workaholics" or "overachievers." For this type of person, production is of prime importance, and little time is spent relaxing. Much like the child who considers a spanking worth the valued attention, some people consider headaches to be worth the reinforcement of attention and promotion. The result? The life-style is unchanged, and headaches continue.

If many headache victims consciously or unconsciously perceive the reinforcement of their life-styles to outweigh the negative consequence, then a potent adversive consequence must consistently occur immediately following the behavior if we hope to see a change in behavior. While headaches certainly qualify as potent adversive consequences, they generally do not occur consistently and do not occur immediately following examples of maladaptive life-styles. When this is the case, psychological theory again predicts that a headache

119

victim will continue avoiding making internal and external changes necessary to modify his or her behavior and way of life.

CONTROL

A major emphasis of the multimodal program for headache relief is *controlling tension*. The importance of this task cannot be overemphasized. Stress and tension are known culprits in the muscle-contraction headaches and are thought by many researchers to play the same role in migraine attacks.

Exactly how stress, social pressure and emotional tensions are translated into muscle tension and headaches is poorly understood. One reason for this is that in traditional medicine and psychology, reactions to stress and tension are considered in terms of the mechanics that cause physiologic changes; consequently, emotional changes or the contributing physiologic causes involved in emotional changes are ignored.

Controlling tension and stress can make a difference in your headache. First, identify the "stressors" in your life. Second, map out a systematic plan to control stress. It is not realistic to think that you can live a totally tension-free life, and, in fact, some tension is good in the sense that it serves to motivate us and keep us alert. Perhaps your environment can be altered in some way to relieve tension.

Controlling diet should also be part of your multimodal plan for headache relief. Appendix A lists foods that the National Migraine Foundation suggests should be avoided by migraine victims. Research suggests dietary factors are associated in about one-third of all migraine attacks.

PRACTICE

Only with consistent and serious practice can the multimodal program for headache relief work for you. This program is designed especially for those headache sufferers who have not received relief from traditional medical treatment.

Relaxation, for example, is a skill that must be developed. Do not make the mistake of assuming that if you are not tense, then you must be relaxed. Like other skills (playing golf or driving a car), relaxation comes with the knowledge of proper technique and practice.

Massage and muscle manipulation must also be practiced consistently, especially since relaxation of the shoulders, neck and facial muscles can prevent the onset of tension. You should become knowledgeable as to which muscles cause you the most problems, and then practice massaging those muscles several times daily. If you have a spouse or other family member willing to assist in the management of your headaches, study Chapter 8 (Massage) together, and practice different massage techniques until you find the one that is most relaxing for you.

Finally, a sensible program of physical conditioning can make a difference in your headaches as well as in your overall health. Start off slowly and practice daily. Remember that twenty or thirty minutes of exercises daily is far better for you than overdoing an hour every three or four days.

RESPONSIBILITY

The multimodal program for headache relief is not intended to substitute for proper medical care but rather to augment it. Rather than being a passive recipient of traditional medical care, assume responsibility for your health by working closely with your physician: Control your diet and the stress in your life, practice relaxation and keep yourself in good physical condition.

Appendix A

Foods to Avoid

Diet has been found to be but one cause of migraine, but some types of foods may actually trigger a headache. The National Migraine Foundation recommends that headache victims avoid the following foods, while taking care to maintain a well-balanced and nutritious diet.

- Ripened cheeses, such as Cheddar, Swiss, Gruyère, Stilton, Brie and Camembert. Suggested alternatives include American, cottage and cream cheeses.
- All fermented, pickled and marinated foods or those containing large amounts of monosodium glutamate, such as bologna, salami, pepperoni and hot dogs.
- Herring, pizza, pork (no more than two to three times per week) and chicken livers.
- Pods of broad beans, such as lima, navy and pea pods; onions and avocados.
- Hot, fresh breads, raised coffee cakes and doughnuts; chocolate.
- Canned figs, citrus foods (no more than one orange per day).
- Vinegar (except white), sour cream, yogurt, nuts, peanut butter and seeds such as sunflower, sesame and pumpkin.
- Excessive tea, coffee, cola beverages (no more than four cups per day) and alcoholic beverages.

Appendix B

Face and Scalp Calisthenics

These exercises can be done several times daily to help relax and tone the muscles of your face and scalp. Get into a habit of practicing these exercises frequently, at work and at home.

- *Eyebrow Stretch.* Lift both eyebrows up towards the hairline as if surprised, and hold them in that position for several seconds. Relax and let the eyes close. Repeat several times.
- *Eye Squint.* Squeeze both eyes into an exaggerated squint, and keep them squinted for several seconds. Relax and let the eyes close. Repeat several times.
- *Mouth Stretch.* Open the mouth as wide as possible (much like yawning). Slowly close the mouth, relax, and repeat the exercise several times.
- *Jaw Stretch.* Open the mouth wide as in the mouth stretch but slide the jaw from right to left and back several times. Relax.
- *Wrinkle Nose.* Wrinkle the nose up in an exaggerated motion as if smelling a very bad odor. Hold this for several seconds, relax, and begin again.
- *Jaw Clench.* Bite down tightly and stretch the corners of the mouth back. Relax and let the jaw drop open. Repeat several times.

Appendix C

Neck and Shoulder Calisthenics

These exercises should be practiced several times daily. It is important to note that they are not intended for muscle development, but they will help loosen and relax your muscles as well as normalize muscle tone. Get into a relaxation habit, practicing the exercises several times throughout each day, as well as when experiencing a headache.

- *Shoulder Lifts.* Raise both shoulders as high as possible in a exaggerated shrug. Relax the trapezius muscles for a moment, and repeat several times.
- *Shoulder Rolls.* Stand or sit with the back straightened, rolling the shoulders in a circular motion for several seconds; rest and repeat.
- *Head Tilt (Left and Right).* Stand or sit with the back straight and slowly tilt the head towards the left shoulder and then over towards the right. Do several times, rest and repeat.
- *Head Tilt (Forward and Back).* Stand or sit with the back straight and slowly drop the chin towards your chest. Slowly raise the chin, allowing the head to drop back as if you were looking at an airplane overhead. Relax and repeat several times.
- *Neck Stretch.* Sit at a desk or table and place either elbow on the table with the palm of the hand against your forehead. Now push your head against your palm; your palm should resist movement. Hold this tension in in the neck for a few seconds and relax.

Index

ergotism, 57
esophagus, 42
ethmoid sinus, 43
eyestrain headaches, 46
face and scalp calisthenics, 123
face massage, 86, 87
feedback loop of pain, 94
food-sensitivity theory, 43, 103, 104–105, 106
foods to avoid, 122
Fothergill, Dr. John, 103
frontalis muscle, 16, 17
frontal lobe, 29
frontal sinuses, 43
fruit, as resistance food, 107
Galen, 10
gate control theory, 27, 28
ginseng, 11
glaucoma, 47
glucose, 110
Griest, Dr. John, 113
hangover headaches, 44, 45
Hanington, Dr. Edda, 104, 105
Harper, A. Murray, 104
"headache personality," 33, 34–35
headache relief, daily plan for, 118–121
headaches, types of, 36–47
    allergy, 43
    brain-tumor, 45, 46
    cluster, 41, 42
    drug-induced, 65
    eyestrain, 46
    glaucoma, 47
    hangover, 44, 45
    hypoglycemia, 42, 110, 111
    ice-cream, 41, 42
    migraine, 39, 40, 41
    sinus, 43, 44
    tension, 36, 37–38, 39
head pain
    history of, 8–12
    surgery for, 68, 69
hemicrania, 10
heterocrania, 10
histamine, 41
Huang Ti, 11
humors. See "temperaments."

hypnosis, 98, 99–101, 102
    components in, 101, 102
    stages of, 99, 100, 101
    uses of, 98, 99
hypoglycemia, 42, 110
    diet for, 111
hypothalamus, 25, 59
ice-cream headaches, 41, 42
involuntary muscles, 24
Jacobson, Dr. Edmond, 96
lysergic acid diethylamide, 59
MAO. See monoamine oxidase inhibitors, 64
massage, types of, 85–92
    acupressure, 90, 91–92
    face, 86, 87
    scalp, 87, 88, 89
    trapezius, 89, 90
maxillary sinuses, 21, 43
medication, 48–65
    analgesic, 49–58, 59
    prophylactic, 58, 59, 60, 61
    psychotropic, 61, 62–64, 65
meditation, 95
Melzack, Dr. Ronald, 27, 28
"meridians," 90
methysergide, 60, 61
migraine
    biofeedback as treatment for, 80, 81, 82
    causes of 26, 39, 40, 41
    description of, 10
    medication for, 55, 56, 57, 60
    theory on, 103, 104, 105, 106
migraine personality, 33, 34–35
migrainous neuralgia. See cluster headache.
monoamine oxidase inhibitors, 64
muscle-contraction headaches. See tension headaches.
muscles
    contraction of, 36, 37–38, 39
    relaxation of, 96, 97, 98
muscles, types of, 16, 17–18, 19
    frontalis, 16, 17
    occipitalis, 16, 17
    temporalis, 16, 17
    trapezius, 18, 19

trigeminal neuralgia, 67
tumor, 45, 46
tyramine, 104, 105, 106
vascular headaches, 15
  causes of, 22, 69
  description of, 80
  medication for, 61
  surgical treatment for, 70

vasoconstriction, 26
vegetables, as resistance food, 106, 107
veins, 13
Volicer, Dr. Beverly J., 33
voluntary muscles, 24
Wall, Dr. Patrick, 27, 28
Wolff, Dr. Harold G., 104